Nursing in Gastroenterology

For Churchill Livingstone:

Commissioning editor: Ellen Green
Project manager: Valerie Burgess
Project development editor: Mairi McCubbin
Design direction: Judith Wright
Project controller: Derek Robertson
Copy editor: Adam Campbell
Indexer: Janine Fearon
Promotions manager: Hilary Brown

Nursing in Gastroenterology

Edited by

Louise Bruce BSc(Hons) MSc RGN PGCEA
formerly Lecturer Practitioner/Senior Nurse, Gastrointestinal Surgery
Oxford Radcliffe NHS Trust, Oxford

Teresa Finlay BSc(Hons) RGN OncCert
Head of Practice Development,
University Hospitals Birmingham NHS Trust, Birmingham

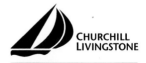

CHURCHILL
LIVINGSTONE

NEW YORK EDINBURGH LONDON MADRID MELBOURNE SAN FRANCISCO AND
TOKYO 1997

CHURCHILL LIVINGSTONE
Medical Division of Pearson Professional Limited

Distributed in the United States of America by Churchill Livingstone, 650 Avenue of the Americas, New York, N.Y. 10011, and by associated companies, branches and representatives throughout the world.

© Pearson Professional Limited 1997

First published 1997

ISBN 0 443 05484 3

British Library Cataloguing in Publication Data
A catalogue record for this book is available from the British Library.

Library of Congress Cataloging in Publication Data
A catalog record for this book is available from the Library of Congress.

Medical knowledge is constantly changing. As new information becomes available, changes in treatment, procedures, equipment and the use of drugs become necessary. The editors/authors/contributors and the publishers have, as far as it is possible, taken care to ensure that the information given in this text is accurate and up to date. However, readers are strongly advised to confirm that information, especially with regard to drug usage, complies with the latest legislation and standards of practice.

The publisher's policy is to use **paper manufactured from sustainable forests**

Printed in the UK by The Bath Press, Bath

Contents

Contributors

Wendy Atkins BSc(Hons)
Ward Sister,
Oxford Radcliffe NHS Trust, Oxford

6 The acute abdomen

Jacqueline Boorman BSc(Hons) SRD
Senior Dietitian in Gastroenterology, Department of Nutrition and
Dietetics, Oxford Radcliffe NHS Trust, Oxford

9 Nutrition

Margaret Butler BN(Hons) RGN RHV
Gastroenterology Specialist / Nurse Practitioner, Royal Liverpool &
Broadgreen University Hospital Trust, Visiting Lecturer, University
of Liverpool, Liverpool

5 Gastrointestinal bleeding

Louise Bruce BSc(Hons) MSc RGN PGCEA
formerly Lecturer Practitioner / Senior Nurse, Gastrointestinal
Surgery Oxford Radcliffe NHS Trust, Oxford

Jill Calvert RGN
Team Leader, Gastrointestinal Surgery, Oxford Radcliffe NHS Trust,
Oxford

6 The acute abdomen

Gina Copp PhD MN DipN(Lond) RGN RCNT
Lecturer in Cancer Care Post-registration Studies Centre for Cancer
and Palliative Care Studies, Institute of Cancer Research, University
of London, Royal Marsden NHS Trust, London

8 Palliative care

Teresa Finlay BSc(Hons) RGN OncCert
Head of Practice Development, University Hospitals Birmingham
NHS Trust, Birmingham

7 Malignancies of the gastrointestinal tract

Susan Goldthorpe RGN
Team Leader, Medical Gastroenterology Unit, Oxford Radcliffe NHS
Trust, Oxford

3 Inflammatory bowel disease

Helen Hamilton RGN
Clinical Nurse Specialist in Parenteral Nutrition, Oxford Radcliffe
NHS Trust, Oxford

9 Nutrition

Jill Hudson BA(Hons) RGN
Team Leader, Surgical Gastroenterology Unit, Oxford Radcliffe NHS
Trust, Oxford

3 Inflammatory bowel disease

Catherine Meadows RGN DipHE
Clinical Nurse Specialist in Stoma Care, Oxford Radcliffe NHS Trust,
Oxford

4 Stoma and fistula care

Elspeth Nesbit BA(Hons) SRN MSc
Formerly Lecturer Practitioner in Palliative Care, Oxford Radcliffe
NHS Trust and Oxford Brookes University, Oxford

8 Palliative care

Catherine Taylor BSc(Hons) RGN
Team Leader, Gastrointestinal Surgery Ward, Oxford Radcliffe NHS
Trust, Oxford

1 Nausea and vomiting
2 Constipation and diarrhoea

Preface

The last decade has seen tremendous changes in health care provision in the United Kingdom. Developing knowledge, skills and technology have all enhanced practice. One of the principal effects of these changes has been the emergence of more specialised areas of practice. In the past, people with gastrointestinal disease were cared for under the umbrellas of 'general medicine' or 'general surgery'. Now there is a clearer recognition of the need to provide specialist nursing care to cater for the needs of these patients. Physical complications and the effects on lifestyle, employment and relationships require expert advice and support through both the acute and the chronic phases of these diseases.

This book aims to help nurture such specialist practitioners by providing the first British text focused entirely on gastrointestinal (GI) nursing. All the contributors are experts in their fields of practice and have provided a rich mix of approaches to nursing patients with particular problems or illnesses. The chapters are not uniform: as no two patients are alike, neither are health care practitioners. Each chapter gives a particular approach to patient care and may be read individually for reference, or as part of the whole.

Despite these differences in approach, all the contributors share the philosophy that the *patient* is absolutely central to practice. As a result, we believe this text differs from others in that its focus is not on gastrointestinal diseases, but on the *people* who suffer from such diseases and on the nursing care that can help to alleviate their suffering. It is not a medically focused gastroenterology book; further reading lists and useful addresses will guide the reader to alternative sources for such information. The intention is to provide a moderate empirical basis of knowledge upon which the moral, ethical and practical aspects of GI nursing can be built.

Real people from everyday practice have been used to illustrate the substance of the text through case studies (their anonymity has, of course, been preserved). These people have been affected by GI disease, not only physically, but in almost every aspect of their lives because of the central role of the digestive system and its related physiology in the maintenance of health and well-being. The overall aim of the book is to provoke thought and stimulate discussion on patient-centred issues that all GI nurses will encounter. Ultimately, we hope that out of the ashes of the 'generic nurse' will come the specialist 'expert gastrointestinal nurse', who will make a significant difference to the lives of those for whom these nurses care.

We would like to thank the contributors for their commitment to this valuable project, and our families and friends for their encouragement and support. Patients and colleagues have motivated us and stimulated our enthusiasm for nursing within this field, and deserve a special acknowledgement as, without them, this book would never have been written.

1997   Louise Bruce
                                                     Teresa Finlay

Nausea and vomiting

Catherine Taylor

INTRODUCTION

The successful management of nausea and vomiting is based primarily on rectifying or minimising the cause, which in turn depends on the pathophysiology of each condition. After careful assessment of an individual's potential and actual experiences of symptoms, the nurse may administer pharmacological measures tailored to the patient's needs and responses. The physiological consequences of symptoms must be minimised, so as to ensure that the patient's health is not compromised further. The nurse has opportunities to provide more than drug administration and practical clinical skills for the management of symptoms. However, in doing so she must ensure that she has the knowledge, accountability and support to demonstrate a commitment to a more human aspect of delivering care. Holistic care has as its emphasis the whole person, rather than the disease/symptom process. It considers health as a state of psychological, social and physical well-being, all of which are intricately interrelated and influencing. Nursing is essentially a caring process which is complementary to, but distinctly separate from, purely medical management.

The symptoms of nausea and vomiting are profoundly psychologically distressing; however their impact is rarely discussed outside the field of chemotherapy. It is from this discipline that gastroenterology nurses may apply and adapt successful measures to their own clinical area.

The experience of nausea plagues gastroenterological conditions, and yet its impact is often overlooked or trivialised. It has been described as having a 'second class status' due to its subjectiveness and to the lack of observable parameters. However, nausea can cause immense psychological distress, often causing isolation and withdrawal from others, and affecting personal coping mechanisms. The nurse can hold the key to unlocking such a psychological impact, by demonstrating genuine empathy and encouraging the use of self-care and behavioural interventions.

Nausea is believed to have a strong psychogenic component. One only has to consider certain English phrases to gain an insight into the link between emotions and nausea. Metaphors involving the gut include 'yellow belly', 'scared sick', 'gutless' and 'butterflies in the stomach'. Accurate and practical techniques for assessing a patient's 'experience' of nausea and vomiting are beset with problems. One tool that may be of some use in qualitatively assessing a patient's perception is the 'Rhodes index' of nausea and vomiting. This requires a patient to rate the frequency, duration and distress suffered from symptoms (Rhodes 1984).

The distress, although probably related to duration and frequency of symptoms, is an extremely personal and unique concept. The use of assessment scales in gastroenterology may be limited, but can ensure that the patient's distress is acknowledged, believed and actively considered by nursing staff.

PATHOPHYSIOLOGY

The symptoms of nausea and vomiting provide a sophisticated 'protective' mechanism. In biological terms, the act of vomiting ensures that toxins or poisons ingested by an individual are forcefully expelled. Vomiting can remove offending or dangerous substances, thus preventing danger and increasing the likelihood of survival.

Nausea both deters further ingestion of substances and halts digestion, thus preventing absorption from occurring before the substances are vomited. Interestingly, nausea can also be associated with the smelling of pungent odours of substances that are 'off', thus preventing substances from being eaten at all (Hawthorn 1995). Within the field of gastroenterology, the symptoms of nausea and vomiting are widespread. In clinical practice their function is often not protective, but a response to a diverse range of underlying conditions, disease states and treatments.

Nausea, retching and vomiting are terms that are often used interchangeably or in tandem but such usage is misleading. Nausea and retching may not culminate in vomiting, and similarly vomiting can occur suddenly and without the 'warning' of nausea. Therefore, the symptoms of nausea, retching and vomiting are more effectively managed by nurses who can define and appreciate the differences.

Nausea

Nausea is a subjective symptom, which is best defined by the individual experiencing it. In practice it is often considered as simply 'feeling sick' or 'wanting to be sick'. A working definition may be: 'the need or desire to vomit, manifested by an unpleasant wave-like sensation in the back of the throat, epigastric and abdominal area' Peters (1989).

The feeling of nausea occurs as a result of changes in the normal regular contraction and relaxation of the stomach. In order to minimise digestion and absorption of unwanted substances, the stomach becomes flaccid, losing its usual gastric tone. Nausea results from the slowing, or sometimes cessation, of gastric motility. The other feature is the reversal of duodenal movement, known as retroperistalsis, whereby the contents of the duodenum are passed back into the stomach, ready to be vomited.

The significance of gastric motility can be experienced simply by eating an excessive amount of rich foods. The fat content reduces gastric motility – hence the well-known feeling of nausea after an overindulgence of cream cakes! Certain drugs, e.g. cisapride, can increase gastric tone and motility; they also have anti-nausea properties but are not necessarily good anti-emetics.

An individual who is experiencing nausea, may exhibit signs of increased sympathetic nervous system activity. The physiological reason for this is unknown. These signs are valuable in assessing nausea in those who are unable or unwilling to report feelings. Individuals may appear pale, cold or clammy and experience cold sweats, and the pulse may rise. It appears that the secretion of gastric acid is decreased and salivation increases. This may be a protective phenomenon, whereby the alkaline saliva can buffer the damaging effect of gastric acid on the oesophagus and mouth.

Retching

Retching is controlled by the respiratory centre in the brain which is also responsible for the changes in rate and depth of respiration observed with the sensation of nausea and the act of vomiting (Hogan 1990). The overall function of retching is unclear, but it is thought that the rhythmic movement may move stomach and duodenal contents to a suitable position for vomiting.

Retching may be thought of as trying to breathe in against a closed glottis. The external intercostal muscles, the diaphragm and the abdominal muscles all contract together, causing an overall decrease in intrathoracic pressure with a concomitant increase in abdominal pressure.

Retching may continue in the absence of vomiting, this distressing phenomenon is commonly known as 'dry heaves'. This may demonstrate an absence of a negative feedback loop, whereby the body cannot detect that the stomach is empty. Overall, it is possible that the number of retches that occur may be related to the nature and volume of gastric contents.

Vomiting

The process of vomiting starts with a deep inspiration. The glottis is then closed to protect the respiratory passages, and air is subsequently drawn into the oesophagus, helping to distend the tube. The soft palate is elevated to prevent vomit entering the nasopharynx. The intercostal muscles and diaphragm contract, and the oesophageal sphincter relaxes. The main expulsive effort is provided by the powerful contraction of the abdominal muscles (rectus abdominus) and the external oblique muscles overlying the stomach. This force on the flaccid stomach and against the negative thoracic pressures causes expulsion of gastric contents through the mouth.

The vomiting reflex

In order to understand the management of nausea and vomiting, it is vital to understand the pathways involved. An understanding based on scientific fact can be applied to nursing care.

The reflex may be divided into three components: detectors, coordinators and effectors. The detectors are responsible for identifying the need to vomit. Unfortunately, detectors are unable to differentiate between poisons, therapeutic drugs or unusual quantities of body constituents, such as breakdown products of tissue damage due to surgical procedures. Therefore, the normally protective symptom can become a useless and distressing symptom during certain conditions, treatments or surgical interventions.

Peripheral pathway detector

The stomach and duodenum have 'chemoreceptors' that respond to ingested substances irritating the mucosal lining, such as bacterial toxins, aspirin or anaesthetic agents. These receptors also respond to conditions which may cause ischaemia or inflammation to the mucosal cells, as in Crohn's disease. The other type of receptors are 'mechanoreceptors', which respond to overdistension or stomach motility changes, such as that resulting from overindulgence in fatty foods or the presence of an obstructing tumour. The detection of these are relayed to the brain via the vagus nerve of the parasympathetic nervous system.

The chemoreceptor trigger zone (CTZ)

The CTZ lies on the surface of the brain stem on the floor of the fourth ventricle; its position is in the area postrema (Fig. 1.1). The zone, despite being located in the brain, is effectively outside the blood–brain barrier and is able to detect emetogenic substances circulating in the blood, such as opiates. The CTZ is also in contact with substances in the cerebrospinal fluid due to its location on the floor of the fourth ventricle.

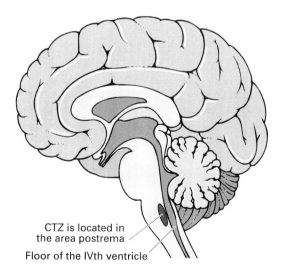

CTZ is located in
the area postrema

Floor of the IVth ventricle

Fig 1.1   The location of the chemoreceptor trigger zone.

Within the field of gastroenterology, the roles of the peripheral gastrointestinal pathway and the CTZ are of paramount importance. However, other pathways are involved in the stimulus to vomit, adding further to this complicated reflex.

The vestibulocerebellar pathway
The vestibulocerebellar pathway involves the labyrinth of the inner ear and the cerebellum. These pathways are stimulated during motion, e.g. during rides at fun fairs, when a rapid change in motion and a difficulty in maintaining orientation through vision can give rise to motion sickness.

The cerebral cortex pathway
The cerebral cortex pathway involves the higher cognitive areas, i.e. the conscious and unconscious self. This may be stimulated by a vast array of senses such as smells, sights, and those of memory, pain and association. Understanding the relevance of this is important for nurse, who has a genuine commitment to holistic care.

Coordinator VC and effectors
The vomiting centre (VC) processes the information received from the above pathways, and orchestrates the complex sequence of events that results in nausea, retching and vomiting. The VC is located in the brain-stem, also on the floor of the fourth ventricle. Once stimulated, the VC initiates events by various outputs: the motor nerves coordinate respiratory muscle movement, the vagal nerves control gastric acid secretion, and sympathetic nerve activity control systemic responses. The processes that occur during vomiting are normal bodily activities; however, during vomiting they are coordinated in such a manner as to ensure that the vomiting reflex results in the expulsion of gastric contents (see Fig. 1.2).

NURSING ASSESSMENT

The foundation of effective nursing care is based on a detailed and ongoing assessment of individual who is at risk of or currently suffering from the symptoms of nausea and vomiting. Central to successful assessment is the ability to communicate. Nurses can promote successful understanding by using language that is mutually understood and which is familiar to the patient. When referring to nausea and vomiting, it may seem more sociable to use medical terms, but these may baffle the patient or be misinterpreted. The nurse benefits from letting patients explain how they are feeling in their own words, and then using these words accordingly. Nausea and vomiting are symptoms that are described with colourful colloquial sayings, such as 'feeling queasy' or 'spewing up'. Their use may be of importance whilst caring for individuals.

Ideally, assessment is carried out on admission and is updated as the patient/nurse relationship develops and the individual's condition/treatment changes. The initial assessment often provides a 'climate' of rapport that can be built on. Therefore, special consideration should be given to

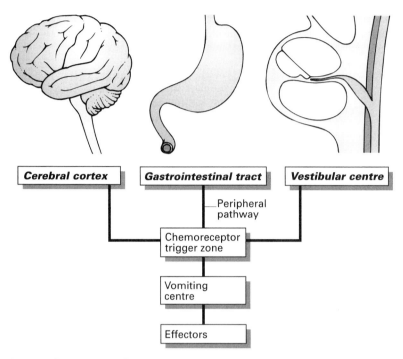

Fig 1.2 The vomiting reflex.

ensuring that adequate time and attention are given to the individual, without distractions. The process of assessment can, in many ways, demonstrate a genuine interest and concern for the individual.

During assessment it is fundamental to review whether the individual is prone to nausea and vomiting under any particular circumstances, e.g. motion sickness, pregnancy, stress or overindulgence. The nurse may then evaluate how any previous experiences were managed and the success of the approaches used. Bad experiences may cause concern for the individual, and the nurse may be able to allay fears and reduce anxiety regarding a repeated experience. Anxiety is thought likely to influence the perception of nausea, but its precise contribution is unknown (Hawthorn 1995).

Overall, the assessment of an individual may give valuable clues about their predisposition to symptoms and/or the variation in the levels at which they experience them. The assessment can enable specific targeting of individuals for prophylactic measures, and a proactive approach to minimising or preventing symptoms. It is, of course, crucial to consider whether pregnancy is a possible cause of nausea in new admissions – this is all too easy to overlook!

Research, mainly in postoperative patients, demonstrates a certain trend in the incidence of nausea and vomiting. The incidence is extremely low in babies and children under 3 years old. An increase occurs after puberty which is more pronounced in females, especially those under 30 years of age. Throughout adulthood the incidence remains fairly stable, although the elderly tend to report a slightly lower incidence.

Gender appears to be highly significant, with reports of women being three times more likely to suffer symptoms than men in the postoperative period (Thompson 1992). This may be correlated to the circulating levels of the female hormone oestrogen. The incidence of symptoms is similar in children of both sexes, but increases in girls as the menarche occurs, and then falls again after the menopause to levels similar to those found in males. Similarly, the timing of the menstrual cycle appears to influence the intensity of symptoms, being more pronounced and likely to occur during menses (Hawthorn 1995).

It has been suggested that individuals who report a history of excessive alcohol intake experience less nausea and vomiting. This blunted response may be due to the chemoreceptor trigger zone being less receptive to an emetic stimulus (Hogan 1990).

It seems that obese individuals experience a higher incidence of postoperative symptoms than thin patients. The reasons are largely unknown, but it is thought that they have a larger proportion of fat in which fat-soluble anaesthetics can dissolve, and require larger doses which take longer to be metabolised, or they have pre-existing medical conditions that may predispose them, e.g. diabetes mellitus. An assessment of previous experiences of post-anaesthesia nausea and vomiting is very useful. This is a commonly expressed fear by patients.

Individuals who are normally susceptible to motion sickness and sickness in pregnancy seem more prone to nausea and vomiting with other disease states or treatments.

The assessment of individuals suffering from nausea and vomiting is best performed by nurses who spend proportionally longer and more intimate time with the individual. The distress and physiological consequence of such symptoms should be relayed to the medical staff, whilst acting as the patient's advocate. The nurse may assist medical investigations if the cause is unknown. Consideration should be given to:

- the patient's medical history and present condition
- an abdominal examination, including the presence or absence of bowel sounds and pain
- a review of past and present drug regimes
- a test of the blood biochemical status
- a rectal examination including digital examination
- a plain abdominal X-ray.

During the assessment period, if the cause of nausea and vomiting is unknown, anti-emetics should not be given as they may mask symptoms and in some cases block the intended 'biological' protective function; for instance, vomiting may have a beneficial effect in food poisoning to eliminate the unwanted substances.

The nurse may gain valuable information for medical diagnosis by making a qualitative assessment of the vomitus including the colour, odour and contents, e.g. pus, mucus, bile, food, gastric secretions. The volume is also important; a large volume may indicate gastric outflow obstruction. If there are small amounts, it may be pertinent to ensure the patient is actually vomiting and not just expectorating. This can be tested by ensuring that the vomit turns blue litmus paper pink due to the presence of gastric acid (Roberts 1993).

Nursing assessment forms the basis for devising individualised care planning, using a problem-solving approach. The assessment provides a framework from which the nurse and patient can devise goals for symptom management and plan care accordingly. During this process, it is essential that there is collaboration with medical staff, colleagues and the patient's family and friends, so as to provide a team approach with a common understanding and aim. Symptom management is rarely straightforward and therefore requires a degree of creativity and expertise in assessing the effectiveness of care.

CAUSES OF NAUSEA AND VOMITING (see Box 1.1)

The symptoms of nausea and vomiting are common. Their aetiology is often multifactorial and influenced by numerous biological, psychological and social variables. The following main conditions will be reviewed with regard to symptoms:

- disorders of the GI tract
- terminal illness
- postoperative nausea and vomiting.

Box 1.1 Causes of nausea and vomiting

1. Intestinal obstruction
    - Fibrous adhesions
    - Intussusception of bowel
    - Sigmoid volvulus
    - Change in intraluminal pressure due to presence of malignant tumour or ulcer
    - External pressure on the bowel, e.g. ovarian tumour
    - Pyloric stenosis

2. Inflammatory processes
    - Gastroenteritis
    - Peritonitis
    - Acute pancreatitis
    - Acute cholecystitis
    - Crohn's disease
    - Hepatitis
    - Appendicitis
    - Peptic ulcer

Box 1.1 (*cont'd*)

3. Motility disorder
   - Non-ulcer dyspepsia
   - Pyloric stenosis
   - Postoperative ileus
   - Constipation
   - Postgastric surgery (dumping syndrome)

4. Irritation
   - Bacterial or viral infection
   - Bacterial toxins in food poisoning
   - Gastric manipulation during surgery/investigations

5. Drug treatment
   - Chemotherapy
   - Anti-Parkinsonian drugs
   - Antidepressants (selective serotonin reuptake inhibitors)
   - Opiate analgesics
   - Anaesthetic agents
   - Digoxin
   - Aspirin
   - Iron
   - Many antibiotics

6. Psychic and neurological factors
   - Raised intercranial pressure
   - Severe pain
   - Unpleasant odours
   - Offensive sights
   - Fear
   - Anxiety
   - Association with a memory

7. Metabolic imbalance
   - Diabetic ketoacidosis
   - Uraemia from renal disease
   - Hypercalcaemia associated with bony metastases
   - Addison's disease

8. Miscellaneous
   - Diseases of the ear e.g. tinnitus or Ménière's disease
   - Migraine
   - Urinary tract infection
   - Motion sickness
   - AIDS
   - Pregnancy
   - Alcohol
   - Spicy foods
   - Self-induced

Vomiting due to disorders of the gastrointestinal tract

Many disorders of the gastrointestinal tract may elicit the vomiting reflex via the peripheral pathway.

Mechanoreceptors and chemoreceptors in the mucosa of the tract respond to inflammation or irritation and relay impulses to the chemoreceptor trigger zone via the vagus nerve. Inflammation of the mucosa may occur in a variety of situations and conditions. The most simple cause is the intake of spicy food and excess alcohol, which may come to light when assessing an individual's dietary and alcohol intake habits. Certain drugs can cause symptoms, e.g. digitalis, antibiotics, aspirin and steroids; they should therefore be taken with or after food to minimise the risk of irritation. Disease-induced nausea and vomiting may occur with conditions such as gastroenteritis, Crohn's, ulceration, appendicitis or the presence of a tumour.

Mechanoreceptors will detect distension of the stomach and small intestine. Whilst this may occur simply with the overindulgence of food, it may indicate the presence of, or compression by, a tumour. Disordered motility in the large bowel and constipation can lead to nausea, but vomiting is uncommon.

Pyloric stenosis can occur when the muscle wall of the pyloric sphincter becomes thickened due to chronic ulceration. The stenosis causes forceful projectile vomiting, which is not associated with the timing of eating and typically contains large volumes of foul-smelling, semi-digested food. Treatment involves surgery to prevent further ulceration and to establish normal gastric function, although sometimes, endoscopic balloon dilatation of the pylorus is sufficient. (Note that this condition should not be confused with pyloric stenosis seen in babies, which is an entirely different condition beyond the scope of this book. Interested readers should refer to a paediatric text.)

Nausea and vomiting in the terminally ill

That the vomiting reflex may be influenced by a multitude of factors is well illustrated by the causes of nausea and vomiting in the terminally ill. The emetic stimulus may come from the disease process, the treatment therapy and/or pre-existing conditions. These may all 'add up' to compound symptoms.

An individual who has a primary tumour of the gastrointestinal tract may have a degree of abdominal distension. This may be compounded by the compression of an enlarged liver due to metastases and the presence of abdominal ascites. The disease may give rise to a variety of conditions such as hypercalcaemia from bony metastases or deranged metabolism caused by hepatic metastases in advanced cancer.

The palliative therapy of a terminally ill patient may involve use of opiate analgesia. For example, morphine has a direct emetogenic action on the CTZ. It also delays gastric emptying and causes constipation, all of which contribute to nausea.

Terminally ill patients may be bedridden, with a low level of bowel motility, a degree of constipation, and periodic urinary tract infections, which may all contribute to feelings of nausea.

Vomiting due to cancer treatments such as radiotherapy and chemotherapy is well known. The gastroenterology nurse may not be directly involved in such care, but may need to give advice and reassurance to patients who have therapy planned. Nurses also need to have an appreciation of how previous therapy may have affected patients, both physically and psychologically, when they are admitted into the gastroenterological unit.

The terminally ill patient may be taking other drugs such as antidepressants which act by inhibiting the reuptake of serotonin (selective serotonin reuptake inhibitors, SSRIs). The raised serotonin levels may cause symptoms of nausea. Anti-Parkinsonian drugs elevate central dopamine levels, and may also contribute to symptoms.

Postoperative nausea and vomiting

Patients undergoing surgery frequently suffer symptoms of nausea and vomiting. The nature of the anaesthetic can influence the severity of symptoms of nausea and vomiting. Spinal anaesthesia and, to a lesser extent, epidural anaesthesia may also cause symptoms. This is often a result of inducing hypotension and a degree of hypoxia. Inhalation anaesthetics such as ether were renowned for their nauseogenic properties; however, now that halothane, and other anaesthetics are used, the incidence of postoperative nausea has reduced considerably.

The maintenance of general anaesthesia is usually achieved by a combination of inhalation and intravenous agents. The emetic action of nitrous oxide has been controversial, but it is thought to share some of the emetic action of the opiates. The gas may also cause symptoms by diffusing into the colon and stomach causing overdistension, whilst at the same time belching and passing flatus are inhibited (Thompson 1992).

The surgical patient may receive analgesia as part of a premedication, peri- and postoperatively. Commonly, opiates such as morphine or Pethidine are administered. Opiate-induced symptoms are a result of the direct effect opiates have on u-opioid receptors on the chemoreceptor trigger zone. The opiates indirectly affect changes in gastric tone and motility, provoking stimulation of peripheral pathways. They also sensitise the labyrinthine apparatus, thus affecting the vestibular pathway. Other drugs used perioperatively that may exacerbate nausea are the opiate derivative fentanyl, neostigmine, used by anaesthetists to reverse muscle relaxants, and metronidazole, an antibiotic commonly given after gut surgery.

During surgery or laparoscopy, the physical handing and manipulation of the gastrointestinal tract will cause stimulation of mechano- and chemoreceptors and massive release of the serotonin from the enterochromaffin cells of the gut mucosa (Thompson 1992). Postoperatively there is a strong likelihood of gastrointestinal stasis or paralytic ileus. The result of reduced gastric motility may be a build-up of gastrointestinal secretions and saliva, the accumulation of which may cause distension and nausea. The distension may need to be relieved by passing a nasogastric tube and allowing free drainage of gastric contents. The nasogastric tube should be left in situ until the gastric motility has resumed, i.e. when bowel sounds can be auscultated.

PHARMACOLOGICAL MANAGEMENT

Preventing or treating the distressing symptoms of nausea and vomiting presents many challenges to nursing practice. Understanding anti-emetic treatment is vital, and flexibility in pharmacological management is the key. The nurse needs to apply knowledge to the judicious selection of the prescribed anti-emetics and make careful evaluation of their effectiveness and possible side-effects.

Anti-emetics comprise a diverse range of drugs, many having been discovered from their use in other aspects of medicine, and some by accident. Historically, gastrointestinal maladies have been treated with a bizarre repertoire of medicines, including blackberry wine, calamis root and five small flint rocks in a glass of water (Jablonski 1993). Present-day pharmacological measures are rather less colourful, but are nevertheless varied and constantly changing.

The optimal choice of an anti-emetic is not simple. Research and clinical trials are fraught with difficulties due to the numerous variables involved. To find the 'best' anti-emetic, efficacy must be related to one standard emetic stimulus, its time duration, route of administration, side-effects and patient response. It is therefore difficult to establish which is the 'best' drug, but the gastroenterology nurse should consider the following factors:

- the underlying cause of the nausea and/or vomiting
- the mechanism by which the anti-emetic works
- the duration of action
- the preferred and optimal route of administration
- patients' preference and individual response
- actual and potential side-effects, especially with long-term use
- availability and cost of medication.

Anti-emetic administration

Anti-emetic treatment should ideally be considered as a prophylactic measure for all patients undergoing treatment that is likely to cause nausea and vomiting, especially for patients who are susceptible. Proactive measures can help prevention or at the least minimise symptoms. Timing of anti-emetic drug administration is vital, in order to maximise their effectiveness. The nurse needs an understanding of their duration of action and may tailor this to certain activities, e.g. by administering prior to getting up postoperatively or before mealtimes.

The route of administration is also important to maximise the effectiveness of the drug and the patient's comfort. A tablet may be inappropriate for a patient who is nauseated, as it may induce vomiting or be vomited before becoming effective. A suppository may be more suitable, but if a patient is actively vomiting, an intravenous or intramuscular injection will have a quicker effect. Syringe drivers can be particularly useful, as constant drug plasma levels can be achieved whilst relieving patients of painful injections. The use of continuous administration occurs mainly in the palliative care setting, where the concern for side-effects is minimal in comparison to the need to control symptoms.

The administration of anti-emetics requires a great deal of thought and thorough evaluation. In many circumstances the complex variety of causes of symptoms may not be relieved by one single anti-emetic. In this case, a combination of drugs with different types of action are more likely to have a positive effect.

Review of anti-emetics (see Table 1.1)

Dopamine receptor antagonists

The majority of anti emetics currently in use are dopamine receptor antagonists. These include metoclopramide, haloperidol, domperidone and prochlorperazine. Their efficacy in controlling nausea and vomiting is a result of the following main actions:

- they antagonise dopamine receptors in the CTZ, involved in the vomiting reflex; and/or
- they affect dopamine receptors in the peripheral pathway, thereby generally increasing peristalsis and decreasing reflux, by facilitating gastric emptying.

The use of dopamine receptor antagonists occasionally causes side-effects,

Table 1.1 Anti-emetic drugs and their uses

Drug classification	Drug	Action	Use
Antihistamine	Cyclizine	Block H_1 receptors of vomiting centre	Motion sickness, bowel obstruction
Anticholinergics	Hyoscine hydrobromide	Antimuscarinic and antispasmodic	Motion sickness, postoperative
Butyrophenones	Droperidol	D_1 receptor antagonist at central CTZ site	Postoperative, uraemia, hypercalcaemia
Substitute butyrophenones	Domperidone	D_1 receptor antagonist at peripheral site	Postoperative
Substituted benzamide	Metoclopramide	Low dose: D_1 receptor antagonist High dose: $5HT_3$ antagonist	Postoperative, opiate-induced symptoms
Phenothiazines	Chlorpromazine Prochlorperazine	D_1 receptor antagonist, peripheral and central effects	Postoperative opiate-induced, metabolic disturbance
$5HT_3$ receptor antagonists	Granisetron Odansetron	$5HT_3$ receptor antagonists, vagus and near CTZ	Chemotherapy and radiotherapy, postoperative

due to dopamine's many actions in the central nervous system. Mild side-effects are related to hypotension, giving rise to faintness and dizziness. In the elderly, this may be compounded by interference with temperature regulation, leading to falls and hypothermia. Some individuals experience restlessness and agitation, often described as the jitters. This is known as 'akathisia', literally meaning the 'inability to sit down'.

More alarming side-effects are a group of symptoms known as extrapyramidal reactions (EPR). These begin with the odd feeling of the tongue swelling (although it isn't) and the jaw locking. The symptoms increase to spasmodic contractions of the neck and facial muscles (torticollis) and spasms of eyeball movement (oculogyric crisis). These are known as acute dystonic reactions. They occur because the extrapyramidal system of the brain is concerned with spinal pathways that control voluntary motor activity and muscle tone. The use of dopamine receptor antagonists can disturb normal dopaminergic pathways of the extrapyramidal tract. Similar disturbances can also be seen in Parkinson's disease.

Side-effects are more common in females, the very young and the very old. They usually occur following excessive doses, or therapeutic doses given on consecutive days.

Butyrophenones–haloperidol, droperidol. These are dopamine receptor antagonists that act centrally in the CTZ. They are used as antipsychotic drugs for conditions such as schizophrenia. Their central action can give rise to a variety of EPRs and pronounced sedative effects.

Intravenous droperidol is often used in postoperative nausea and vomiting. However, postoperative recovery from anaesthesia can be significantly delayed by its effects (Rowbottom 1992). Hence droperidol can be used in the acute phase as a 'one-off' dose, in conjunction with opiate analgesics via an infusion pump. Haloperidol is often used in combination therapy in the palliative care setting.

Substituted butyrophenones–domperidone (Motilium). This dopamine receptor antagonist acts mainly at peripheral sites–hence the lower incidence of EPRs. It acts by improving gastric motility and tone, and is therefore suitable for postoperative nausea and vomiting. However, it is only available in oral and suppository form, as the intramuscular route has been shown to be ineffective, and intravenous use has been withdrawn after its association with cardiac arrhythmias. It is not recommended for long-term administration.

Substituted Benzamide–metoclopramide (Maxalon). Metoclopramide is widely used in treating a variety of functional and organic gastrointestinal disorders that give rise to symptoms of nausea and vomiting. At low doses, it antagonises dopamine receptors, but at high doses it is a $5HT_3$ receptor antagonist. Hence, its use in low dosages for postoperative nausea and vomiting and gastrointestinal disturbances, and in high dosages for radiotherapy and chemotherapy-induced emesis.

Metoclopromide affects gastric motility by improving the tone and peristalsis of the stomach, enabling accelerated gastric emptying, and accelerated transit through the duodenum and jejunum. This property is extremely useful in emergency situations for emptying the stomach prior to anaesthesia. The prophylactic measure can greatly reduce the likelihood of vomiting and aspiration during induction. Because of the effects on motility, it is vital that the nurse does not administer metoclopramide when a condition exists whereby increased motility may be hazardous. Examples of this are when there is a high risk of haemorrhage or perforation, or where an obstruction is present. In some cases it is contraindicated after abdominal surgery.

The effectiveness of metoclopramide in low doses is still under debate. Approximately 50% of studies have shown that it is no more effective than a placebo (Rowbottom 1992). The effects of metoclopramide do, however, seem to be optimum when given towards the end of an operation. High-dose metoclopramide in the oncology setting is usually given as a continuous rather than intermittent infusion to maintain steady plasma levels. Its use, however, is declining with the new range of $5HT_3$ receptor antagonists.

Side-effects with metoclopramide are usually mild, transient and readily reversed by withdrawal of the drug. Common side-effects are sedation, diarrhoea and dizziness. EPRs may occur in those undergoing high-dose treatments, and who are susceptible. Reactions may be treated with procyclidine or diazepam (Pinder 1976).

Phenothiazines–prochlorperazine (Stemetil), perphenazine (Fentazin), chlorpromazine (Largactil). These anti-emetics are widely used, but are often limited by their toxicity, causing, for example, EPRs, hypersensitivity, hormonal dysfunction and sedation. Prochlorperazine is widely used in postoperative nausea and vomiting, and is seen to be effective in reducing opiate-induced symptoms.

Phenothiazines can be useful in treating vertigo, Ménières disease and migraine-induced symptoms (Pinder 1976).

Antihistamines – cyclizine, dymenhydrinate, cinnarizine

This group of drugs act directly on the H_1 receptors of the vomiting centre by antagonising the action of histamine. They appear to be important in the vestibular pathway of the vomiting reflex, and are therefore particularly useful when motion provokes symptoms. Most over-the-counter preparations for travel sickness are antihistamines. Their main drawback is their sedative effect.

Antihistamines have been advocated as the anti-emetic of choice when bowel obstruction, haemorrhage or perforation is suspected, so as to avoid the use of dopamine antagonists which increase bowel motility and may cause complications.

Cyclizine works rapidly and is effective for up to 6 hours. Side-effects are blurred vision, dryness of the mouth and urinary hesitancy. Caution must be taken when nursing patients with respiratory disease as antihistamines can increase the viscosity of lung secretions.

Anticholinergics – Hyoscine hydrobromide

This range of drugs has been isolated from a rather unusual source, the plant *Belladonna alkaloides*, otherwise known as 'deadly nightshade'. The drugs have antimuscarinic activity, with a depressant action on the vomiting centre and an antispasmodic action on the gastrointestinal tract. They are commonly given with premedication, in order to dry bronchial and salivary secretions. Their side-effects are dilation of the pupils, dry mouth, urinary retention and drowsiness. Hyoscine and atropine are used in motion sickness and are frequently used in surgery as part of a premedication regime, for their effects on secretions and their anti-emetic properties. These drugs are avoided in the elderly, who are particularly susceptible to the central anticholinergic side-effects of disorientation and dizziness, as well as glaucoma or urinary retention.

Steroids – prednisolone, dexamethasone

The anti-emetic action of these drugs is still unclear; suggestions include the inhibition of prostaglandin release, the stabilisation of cell membranes and the decrease of the permeability of the blood–brain barrier. Predominantly, their use as an anti-emetic has been within the field of chemotherapy, in a combination regime. They also have a particular role in the treatment of refractory nausea or vomiting, such as may occur in palliative care. Side-effects to look out for include transient glucose intolerance, fluid retention, Cushingoid features, vaginal or anal burning on administration, effects on mood, and insomnia. Long-term usage is inadvisable due to the effects on the immune system (Mitchelson 1992).

Sedatives and anxiolytics – lorazepam, diazepam

These medications are sometimes useful in combination with other anti-emetics. It is debatable whether they actually have any anti-emetic properties, but rather sedative, anxiolytic and amnesic effects that lessen the intensity of nausea and vomiting, making the symptoms more tolerable.

They are of significant value when nausea and vomiting have a strong psychogenic element to them, e.g. during severe anxiety, association nausea.

Cannabinoids – nabilone (Cesamet)

These drugs are derived from the Indian hemp plant (cannabis) from which marijuana is obtained. Their anti-emetic action was noted in the USA when patients who were regular users of cannabis were noted to have a low incidence of nausea and vomiting after chemotherapy (Hawthorn 1995). The action of nabilone is still unknown, but it has been found to be effective in treating unresponsive vomiting due to cytotoxic drugs. Its use within gastroenterology is limited, especially with unfavourable side-effects such as hallucinations, hypotension and dizziness.

Nabilone is a semi-synthetic cannabinoid, used in chemotherapy-induced nausea and vomiting, designed specifically to be an anti-emetic. Its positive effects are mood elevation and reduced pain recognition. (Note that cannabis is not a licensed drug; its supply and use is illegal under all circumstances in the UK).

The 5HT₃ receptor antagonists – ondansetron, granisetron, tropisetron

The neurotransmitter serotonin, or $5HT_3$, is found in its highest concentration in the enterochromaffin cells of the gut mucosa. It has a wide variety of actions depending on the conditions and its concentration. $5HT_3$ receptors play a major role in the perception of pain, sleep, anxiety, aggression and migraine and in the nausea and vomiting reflex.

The use of cytotoxic therapy, the manipulation of the gut during surgery or the very act of vomiting releases large amounts of $5HT_3$. $5HT_3$ receptors are thought to activate the vagal nerve, and possibly the vomiting centre. The $5HT_3$ receptor antagonist anti-emetics are designed to block the $5HT_3$ receptors, thus stopping peripheral pathway transmission and central processing. The excellent control of symptoms possessed by these anti-emetics demonstrates the importance of this molecule in the nausea and vomiting reflex. These new anti-emetics have revolutionised symptom control with chemotherapy and radiotherapy patients. Their potential use within gastroenterology looks extremely promising.

The anti-emetics are easily administered either by mouth or intravenously, with only minimal side-effects reported such as headache and mild constipation. They do not act on dopamine receptors and are therefore ideal for the very young and old, who are susceptible to extrapyramidal reactions.

The $5HT_3$ receptor antagonist, ondansetron, has been licensed for use in the prevention and treatment of postoperative nausea and vomiting. It has no effect on anaesthetic recovery time, nor does it induce respiratory depression. At present, its only limitation appears to be cost. However, its success suggests that it will continue to be used and may prove to be the anti-emetic 'wonder drug' of the future (Ploster 1991).

NURSING MANAGEMENT OF NAUSEA AND VOMITING

The effective management of symptoms requires a thorough understanding of the pathophysiology of causes and a framework of assessment from which nursing strategies may be devised. Excellence in clinical practice begins with the use of research-based, scientific knowledge, coupled with the delivery of holistic care.

Nursing management can be planned in a systematic, individualised manner, by using a problem-solving approach. The plan may include potential problems, which fosters a proactive management style, while actual problems call for immediate reactive management. Both require considered nursing interventions which are goal-centred.

Fundamental to the nursing process is the ability to evaluate the outcome of interventions and to adjust management according to their success or failure.

Review of potential/actual symptom problems

Potential/actual problem of dehydration

In solving this problem, the aim is to restore normal fluid and electrolyte balance. The assessment questions are:

- Are they showing signs and symptoms of dehydration?
- Is there physiological fluid or electrolyte imbalance?
- What hydration support do/may they need?

A patient who is simply nauseated may be reluctant to drink for fear of increasing the nausea or actually vomiting. The nurse must realise the potential for dehydration, explain this to the patient and encourage the oral intake of fluids. The nauseated patient may have a particular preference for a drink; many like fizzy or iced drinks. Ginger ale is an old favourite for relieving gastric disturbances; its extract 6-gingerol is considered to have anti-emetic properties. The initial assessment of mild dehydration is quite difficult, with thirst being the first sign. If the patient has a poor fluid intake (less than 2 L/24 h) or is actually vomiting, a fluid balance chart should be kept. By recording all fluid input and output, the nurse has quantitative evidence of actual or potential fluid and electrolyte imbalance. Daily weight can give a good indication of the fluid balance; for example, with prolonged reluctance to drink and/or vomiting, the fluid balance will be negative, and the patient will lose weight. The patient may exhibit signs and symptoms of dehydration. These include:

- decrease in urine output
- elevated blood levels of urea and electrolytes
- dry furrowed tongue
- decreased skin turgidity
- increased temperature
- fatigue
- deterioration in mental processes.

The patient who is vomiting is at risk of metabolic alkalosis, due to the loss of hydrogen ions $[H^+]$ in gastric acid. The pH of the body rises towards 8.0. The patient can become severely dehydrated and depleted of Na^+ and CL^- ions, a condition known as hypochloreaemic alkalosis. The kidney tries to compensate by conserving H^+, but this occurs at the expense of $[K^+]$ potassium ions. Patients may become hypokalaemic, not only from excess urinary loss but also because of K^+ shift into the cells in response to the alkalosis. The clinical signs of this are fatigue, muscle cramps, irregular pulse and shallow slow respiration, as alkaline plasma depresses the respiratory centre. Signs may be compounded by a patient displaying irrational and irritable behaviour. The patient requires intravenous fluid and electrolyte replacement therapy, as determined by the blood biochemical status (Clancy & McVicker 1992).

The hydration support of patients is an integral part of nursing care. The nurse helps to ensure that the choice of fluid infusate is tailored to the physiological disturbance of the patient suffering nausea and/or vomiting. In general, all infusions should be administered so as to maintain normal body fluid compartment volumes and compositions, in order to achieve normal cellular function or homeostasis. All are infused intravenously, hence into the extracellular fluid, but their dispersal and action depend on their nature. Sodium chloride (normal saline) is an isotonic solution that will distribute throughout all extracellular fluids, and therefore be useful to compensate for lack or loss of fluid. Glucose solutions (dextrose 5%) act similarly but the glucose can actually penetrate cells and eventually be metabolised, enabling intracellular hydration to occur. Both are useful when electrolyte balance is normal, but water balance is disturbed, such as with a patient who is unable to maintain intake due to nausea but who is not actively vomiting. Care must be taken to avoid using dextrose-saline alone since this contains too little sodium for the patient, who may end up hydrated but hyponatraemic. Alternating sodium chloride and glucose infusions are indicated when there is combined water and sodium depletion, such as during persistent vomiting. Potassium concentrations may become deranged during vomiting. The addition of potassium is usually required, to avoid or correct hypokalaemia (Clancy & McVicker 1992).

Potential/actual problem of malnutrition due to vomiting and nausea

The aim is to prevent malnourishment and to ensure satisfactory dietary habits for the patient. The assessment questions should be:

- What is their weight, and have they incurred recent weight loss and why?
- Are they clinically malnourished?
- How do they feel about eating?

A patient who is nauseated and/or vomiting is unlikely to have an appetite. They may become nutritionally depleted, to a greater extent than their gastroenterological condition or treatment actually warrants. This may be exacerbated by periods of fasting prior to investigations, anxiety or unappetising hospital food.

Careful assessment is fundamental to managing this particular problem. A baseline weight and nutritional assessment in liaison with the dietician is invaluable for planning care (see Chapter 9). The patient's likes and dislikes should be recorded, including special dietary requirements for medical, religious or social reasons. The individual's perception of eating provides valuable insight into their anxiety in inducing nausea or vomiting, and other factors that may deter them from eating.

Many psychological factors are involved when considering dietary habits. Patients often feel unable to eat in bed or near their bedside, or near fellow patients who may be expectorating, vomiting or in fact defaecating behind curtains in the same room. The surrounding vomit bowls, urinals, drainage tubes, drips and equipment may all deter or diminish a desire to eat. The nurse should consider, and as far as possible improve, the eating environment for patients.

The timing of meals and interventions may also be important. The prophylactic use of an anti-emetic prior to meals may enhance eating, as may an appetite stimulant such as a measure of sherry. Meals should be light, small and nutritious, and if possible easily stored so that they can be eaten when the patient prefers. Food should have minimal odour and not be highly seasoned or greasy, as fatty foods tend to slow gastric emptying. Practical measures include allowing steam and odour to escape from the food before serving.

Patients should be advised to eat slowly and in a comfortable, suitable eating position. A quiet, undisturbed environment and a rest period after eating may lessen the likelihood of symptoms. When meals are refused, nutritious drinks should be offered. If there is a serious nutritional deficit, the use of enteral or total parenteral nutrition may need to be considered.

Potential/actual problem of inability to care for personal and environmental hygiene

The goal in dealing with this problem is to ensure a high standard of hygiene and suitable environmental conditions for a patient suffering nausea and vomiting. The nurse can play a very creative role in ensuring that a patient distressed by symptoms has maximum privacy, and that attention is given to simple issues that may promote comfort and well-being.

The environment should be considered; both nausea and vomiting are very private phenomena and the thought of being sick in front of others can be extremely distressing. The nurse should manipulate resources to ensure privacy, without compromising safety. The use of side rooms for vulnerable patients is preferable, without causing undue isolation. Leaving the door open, provision of a buzzer and regular checking can provide privacy and quiet, whilst maintaining reassurance with the nurse's presence.

There should be easy access to a receiver and tissues; this is both a reassuring measure and a practical one to minimise soiling. After vomiting, all receivers should be promptly disposed of, after the nature of the vomitus has been assessed and the volume measured.

A mouthwash of the patient's preference should be encouraged to promote comfort and to provide a preventative measure against oral mucosal infection such as *Candida albicans*. After a vomiting episode, efforts should be made to remove all soiled bedclothes and linen, using the usual precautions for handling body fluids. Hand and face washing facilities should be offered to improve feelings of comfort. The vomiting episodes can exacerbate feelings of dirtiness and disturbed body image; by providing simple measures of comfort, the nurse can reduce such negative feelings.

The post-vomiting phase causes a profound feeling of weakness, where individuals can experience muscular aches, pains and feelings of cold and shivering. This severe weakness is poorly understood and is probably more than a reflection of the energy used during the vomiting period. Overall, the provision of rest and adequate sleep is an essential part of the patient's well-being and symptom management. The nurse can strive to promote such rest by actively encouraging periods during which a patient is undisturbed by staff or visitors. Studies have shown that tiredness and sleep deprivation are the most common precipitating factors for nausea in women with morning sickness (Jablonski 1993). In some cases, the temporary use of sedatives to promote rest, and reduce restlessness and anxiety may be necessary.

Management of potential/actual complications of nausea and vomiting

The aim is to recognise and minimise the occurrence of complications, such as:

- exacerbation of discomfort and pain
- potential risk of inhalation of vomit
- potential risk of wound dehiscence due to forceful vomiting
- risk of reduced mobility and inherent problems due to symptoms.

The perception of discomfort and pain within gastroenterological conditions is often coupled with feelings of nausea and the stress of vomiting. The link is twofold – pain is a stimulus known to contribute to nausea and sometimes vomiting, whereas opiates used to relieve pain are themselves emetogenic. It is essential that the nurse anticipates the need for an appropriate and effective combination of analgesics and anti-emetics, tailoring their administration accordingly. Non-emetic analgesics should be considered as appropriate alternatives.

First-line prophylactic care in patients undergoing surgery is to withhold food and drink prior to surgery so as to minimise the risk of vomiting and aspirating during induction of anaesthesia and endotracheal intubation. Basic physiology demonstrates that 4–6 h of starvation is the maximum desirable. Research suggests that patients are often starved for longer periods, as part of a ritualistic approach which involves starving all pre-operative patients from midnight. A more rational action would be to starve for 4–6 h, working back from the scheduled time of operation (Walsh & Ford 1989). Prophylactic measures can include the administration of an anti-emetic as a premedication before surgery.

The unconscious patient is at particular risk of inhaling vomit whilst the cough reflex is inhibited or depressed. They should be nursed with the head down and to one side, with easy access to suction equipment. Inhalation of vomit can give rise to aspiration pneumonitis, whereby the chemical inflammation causes bronchospasm, pulmonary oedema, and respiratory and circulatory collapse (Dunn & Rowlinson 1992).

The effects of forceful retching and vomiting can potentially cause pain or disruption of wound sites, since gastrointestinal surgery often necessitates a large midline incision. The use of a firm support in the form of a cushion or the patient's hand can be helpful in preventing strain on the healing area. Vomiting may rarely cause tears in the mucosa of the lower oesophagus or gastric cardia (Mallory Weiss tear) resulting in a haematemesis, especially in patients who have a history of alcohol abuse or persistent vomiting.

The patient who is feeling nauseated may find that movement exacerbates symptoms, especially when moving from lying flat to standing, since postural hypotension is known to increase nausea. The patient may prefer to remain flat and immobile, and in doing so incurs the risks of prolonged bed rest, such as deep vein thrombosis or pressure sore development. The nurse may preempt this situation by ensuring prophylactic use of anti-emetics prior to mobilisation. Sitting on the side of the bed for a certain period prior to standing, so as to minimise the occurrence of postural hypotension, can be of value. Explanations and assurance that the nausea should subside should be given as appropriate.

NURSING AND SELF-CARE

The use of self-care practices in the management of nausea and vomiting has had sparse attention, except in the field of chemotherapy. Self-care has been suggested as a means of promoting more successful symptom control, and as a way of handing control of a situation over to a patient. Individuals coping with nausea and vomiting must deal with a new set of demands not to be found in their usual repertoire of knowledge and skills (Richardson 1991).

The concept of taking responsibility for one's own care is harnessed with a wide range of meanings that must stimulate a change in attitudes, values and beliefs in traditional nursing practice. With self-care, the emphasis shifts from a custodial role – the 'caring' or 'doing for' which is often deemed the creator of dependence – to a role of 'caring about', which suggests an 'interest for and enablement' of the patient, i.e. a creator of self-determination. Overall, the use of self-care in symptom management should foster support and assistance, rather than control and directing of patients.

Within gastroenterology, the nurse–patient relationship can be complementary, to enable self-care activities; such as self-medication, relaxation / distraction techniques, managing of the environment and activities, and the use of psychological and social support. Before initiating self-care activities, the nurse should consider their appropriateness. For example, it would be inappropriate for the critically ill postoperative patient, but appropriate for a patient with bowel cancer hoping to be discharged home to manage symptoms as independently as possible. Personal motivation, attitude, confidence and support networks should all be considered.

After gaining an insight into the patient's perception and physical abilities, the nurse can plan and implement the teaching of essential knowledge and skills which are a prerequisite for practising self-care.

Self-medication is a programme whereby patients are responsible for their own drug administration in the hospital setting. For controlling nausea and vomiting, the patient is in an ideal position to self-administer anti-emetics at the most appropriate times, especially as a prophylactic measure before activities known to trigger symptoms. This is particularly true in the field of chemotherapy, as the symptoms of nausea and vomiting are often protracted, which is rarely the case in postoperative nausea and vomiting. To initiate self-medication, a formal assessment of the patient's suitability should be carried out, and informed written consent should be obtained. The nurse can facilitate teaching and supervision, as self-care can only be achieved with sufficient knowledge and skill. Patients must understand the correct use of their drugs, their effects for symptom control and, most importantly, their potential side-effects. The goal is for comprehension of and compliance to an anti-emetic regime, which may ultimately enable symptoms to be managed upon patients' discharge into the home. When commencing self-medication programmes, the nurse must be sensitive to patients' deep-seated expectations of the nurse's role. Studies have shown that many patients favour nurses administering their medication, as it complies with the 'usual routine' and they have faith in a nurse's knowledge (Thomas 1992).

Self-medication therefore requires a full explanation and an appropriate introduction to patients and their families, emphasising that it is a means of promoting a patient's independence and control.

Acupressure self-care

An interesting and rather unusual self-care intervention for nausea and vomiting is the use of acupressure bands. The traditional Chinese treatment was first promoted by Professor N. Dundee who had watched women in a Chinese maternity hospital press their right wrist as a means of preventing morning sickness. The relevant point for the control of nausea and vomiting is in the P_6 or Neikuan point, which is approximately 5 cm from the distal wrist crease. This meridian is thought to link the area on the skin to internal organs related to the vomiting reflex. Numerous studies have been performed to demonstrate the use of acupuncture and acupressure on symptom relief, with many demonstrating benefits greater than that of 'dummy' acupressure points. The studies have often been carried out on small groups, and controversy exists about whether symptom relief is due to a patient's belief in the technique or whether there is direct physiological action (Stannard 1989).

Acupressure is a non-invasive procedure for applying pressure, in contrast to the manual needling of an acupuncture point. Specialist wrist bands have been developed commercially, incorporating a stud which, when pressed, can be used over the P_6 point. These are known as 'sea bands' because they were originally used for sea sickness. The patient can self-administer the antiemetic effect by applying pressure for 2–5 min every 2–6 h. Despite the debate surrounding its effects, the use of acupressure can be an excellent, simple and harmless self-care intervention where the patient has an active involvement in symptom control.

The nurse and patient may manage certain aspects of symptoms by paying attention to the simple issues of comfort, well-being and psychological control. These caring practices are non-invasive measures. They require creativity from the nurse and self-care motivation from the patient. Many of the interventions have limitations and should be considered as complementary to, rather than instead of, medical management. At present, there is little research and negligible data to confirm the effectiveness of supportive techniques. Thus, their usefulness must be considered only after evaluating each individual's response to the techniques and the perception of their success.

The nurse and patient may minimise symptoms by the use of patient self-care distraction techniques, which do not necessarily reduce symptoms, especially nausea, but merely 'supersede' them perceptually. Examples of activities that interest and absorb attention include television, games, reading, changes in environment, and listening to music. Above all, the simple presence of a nurse or loved ones who can share time and provide company with interest and humour is invaluable. Music therapy has been found to relax patients and reduce symptoms, with music chosen according to the patient's particular tastes (Ouverkerk 1994).

Most self-care distraction techniques emphasise the need to reduce anxiety and induce relaxation, thus creating a 'state of relative freedom, from both anxiety and skeletal muscle tension, inducing a quieting or calming of the mind' (Watson 1991). The relaxation process is a hypothalamic response that leads to a reduction in activity of the sympathetic nervous system. It is thought that this may interrupt the physiological arousal of the vomiting centre.

Relaxation may be induced simply by the touch of an individual who is concerned and who intends to help the patient. However, touch needs to be tailored to what is personally and culturally acceptable to the patient. Therapeutic touch may involve simply holding the patient's hands, providing support and reassurance and reducing the sense of loneliness while they are suffering from nausea and vomiting. Touch may be performed in a more structured manner such as gentle massage, possibly using aromatherapy oils. Relaxation therapy should preferably be performed in a quiet, undisturbed environment. The patient can be taught to progressively tense and relax different muscle groups, in order to induce low levels of tension. The patient can focus on slow rhythmic breathing, with the use of guided imagery (visualisation) which involves concentrating on pleasant images (Wilson 1988).

Anxiety is thought to contribute to the distress caused by symptoms of nausea and vomiting. The nurse plays a unique role in assessing individuals' anxieties, and throughout their care can help them to address these worries and fears. By providing information regarding their condition, treatment and symptoms, many myths and misconceptions can be dispelled. Research has demonstrated that giving information to a pre-operative patient reduces stress and anxiety and in turn has beneficial effects on postoperative recovery rates (Hayward 1975). Patients have often been subject to overexaggerated horror stories and therefore need reassurance and an explanation of what to expect and what, in terms of symptoms, is usual and commonplace. The nurse can demonstrate respect for each individual by spending time listening to their feelings and their personal experiences. This commitment to listening provides the foundation of the support that individuals need, enabling them to draw on effective coping mechanisms such as self-care activities.

CONCLUSION

Within the field of gastroenterology, the symptoms of nausea and vomiting are common. The gastroenterology nurse plays a crucial intermediary role between the patient and medical management. The nurse can provide optimal management through an understanding of the pathophysiology of causes and symptoms, and by tailoring pharmacological measures accordingly. However, the nurse can offer far more comprehensive management by providing a creative 'human' side to clinical practice. This care embraces the concept of 'holism' and the promotion of self-care. In doing so, the nurse demonstrates respect and value for the intrinsic worth of each patient and their well-being.

REFERENCES

Clancy J, McVicker A J 1992 Which infusate do l need? Professional Nurse June: 586–589

Dunn C D, Rowlinson N 1992 Surgical diagnosis and management. Blackwell Scientific Publications, Oxford, p 38

Hawthorn J 1995 Understanding and management of nausea and vomiting. Blackwell Scientific, Oxford

Hayward J 1975 Information: a prescription against pain. RCN, London

Hogan C M 1990 Advances in the management of nausea and vomiting. Nursing Clinics of North America 25(2):475–493

Jablonski R S 1993 Nausea – the forgotten symptom. Holistic Nursing Practice 65–71

Mitchelson F 1992 Pharmacological agents affecting emesis. A review article. Drugs 43(3):295–315

Ouverkerk A 1994 Cancer therapy – Induced emesis, the nurses perspective. European Journal of Cancer Care 3, p 18–25

Peters C 1989 Myths of antiemetic administration. Cancer Nursing 12(2):102–106

Pinder R M 1976 Metoclopramide; A review of its pharmacological properties and clincial use. Drugs 12:81–131

Ploster L G 1991 Granisetron – a review of its pharmacological properties and therapeutic use as an anti emetic. Drugs 42(5):805–824

Rhodes V A 1984 Development of reliable and valid measures of nausea and vomiting. Cancer Nursing 25: February:33

Richardson A 1991 Theories of self care. Journal of Advanced Nursing 16: 671–676

Roberts A 1993 The management of nausea and vomiting in advanced cancer. Care of the Critically Ill 9(2):64–65

Rowbottom D N 1992 Current management of post-operative nausea and vomiting. British Journal of Anaesthesia 69 (suppl. 1):46–59

Stannard D 1989 Pressure prevents nausea. Nursing Times 85(4): p 33, 34

Thomas C 1992 Reviewing attitudes to self medication. Nursing Times 88(24):50

Thompson J (1992), Post-operative nausea and vomiting. British Journal of Theatre Nursing Oct:22–24

Walsh M, Ford P 1989 Nursing rituals research and rational action. Heinmann Nursing, Oxford

Watson 1991 Cancer patient care – psychosocial treatment methods. Cambridge University Press, Cambridge

Wilson 1988 Nursing issues and research in terminal care. John Wiley, vol 6, ch 8, p 163

FURTHER READING

Burkitt H G, Gait D, Quick 1994 Essential surgery: problems, diagnosis and management. Churchill Livingstone, Edinburgh

Eburm E 1989 Choosing the right anti emetic. Nursing Times 85(24):36–37

Harrington R A 1983 Metoclopramide – an updated review of its pharmacological properties. Drugs 25: 451–494

Pervan V 1993 Understanding anti-emetics. Nursing Times 89(10):36–37

Constipation and diarrhoea

Catherine Taylor

■ CONTENTS

INTRODUCTION

The symptoms of constipation and diarrhoea are common in gastroenterology. The nurse plays a pivotal role in assessing and managing the symptoms, in order to minimise their physiological impact and to prevent complications from occurring. Nursing management can provide care for those whose symptoms cause immense 'psychosocial' problems, and education for those whose symptoms may be managed independently.

Irritable bowel syndrome (IBS) will also be addressed in this chapter as it is characterised by altered, unpredictable bowel habit. Functional gut disorders such as IBS account for approximately 60% of GI outpatient consultations. GI nurses in conjunction with gastroenterologists in outpatients have a vital role to play in helping the patient to manage the condition.

ANATOMY AND PHYSIOLOGY OF THE LARGE INTESTINE

The large intestine begins at the ileocaecal sphincter and terminates at the anus. The colon is divided into the caecum and the ascending, transverse, descending and sigmoid colon, which joints the rectum at the rectosigmoid junction. The muscle wall consists of an outer longitudinal layer and an inner circular layer. The rectum is about 13 cm in length and totally sheathed in a longitudinal muscle layer. Its interior is divided by three circular muscles producing shelf-like folds called the rectal valves.

The colon and rectum are lined with epithelial cells that have crypts but no villi, and many mucus-producing goblet cells. The anal canal has sensitive squamous epithelial cells in continuity with the perineum. The anal canal is 2–5 cm in length and has an internal and an external sphincter (see Fig. 2.1).

The main functions of the large intestine are outlined below:

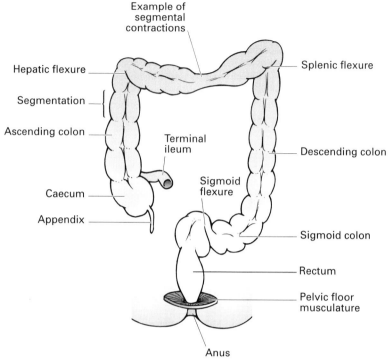

Fig 2.1   Anatomy of the large intestine.

- absorption of fluid and electrolytes
- mixing and propelling contents from the terminal ileum towards the anus
- storage of undigested remnants prior to defaecation
- production of mucus to facilitate the passage of faeces
- harbouring of colonic bacteria for the breakdown of complex carbohydrates and synthesis of vitamins B and K
- absorption of short chain fatty acids.

Large intestine motility

Motility in the large intestine is mediated by its own intrinsic nerve plexus, under the influence of hormones and neurotransmitters such as cholecystokinin, vasoactive intestinal peptide and catecholamines, in addition to the extrinsic nerve plexus. The two main patterns of motility are segmentation and mass movements.

Segmentation contractions occur every 2–3 min; there is a contraction and relaxation of alternate bands of circular muscle, giving a mixing action. Mass movements occur two to three times per day and have a propulsive effect. The strong sweep is usually precipitated by the entry of food into the stomach. This 'gastrocolic' reflex results in peristalsis, driving contents up to 30 cm under relatively high pressures towards the rectum. The overall time for movement from mouth to anus is referred to as the intestinal transit time.

Absorption of fluid and electrolytes

The process of colonic absorption occurs at the mucous membrane, assisted by segmentation motility, which enables greater exposure of contents to the absorptive surface. Approximately 2 L of fluid passes the ileocaecal valve each day, with absorption occurring mainly on the right side of the colon; only about 150 ml is passed in the faeces. Overall, the greater the mixing, the greater is the reabsorption of fluid, with the potential for dehydration of faeces and an increased likelihood of constipation. On the other hand, a 10% reduction in colonic absorption will double the amount of faecal water and result in diarrhoea.

Normal faeces have a water content of 60–80%. The solid matter is made up of approximately 30% bacteria, 2–3% nitrogen, 20% fat and 20% inorganic material. Normal faeces are brown due to the presence of modified bile pigments.

Mechanism of defaecation

Defaecation is the term applied to the expulsion of faeces from the rectum. The rectum is usually empty and collapsed until just before defaecation. When faeces enter, the rectum is passively distensible and acts as an evacuable reservoir. It is very sensitive to a rise in pressure and can discriminate between the presence of solids and gas. The entry of faeces causes local distension and pressure, which gives rise to sensory impulses that lead to relaxation of the internal anal sphincter. The anorectal angle straightens, thus decreasing the acute angle between the rectum and the anal canal. The contraction of the diaphragm and abdominal wall further empty the contents of the left colon into the rectum. When conditions permit, the puborectalis muscles and external anal sphincter relax under voluntary control. This voluntary inhibition controlled by the higher centres of the brain can be learnt by a child at $1-1\frac{1}{2}$ years old, when the pathways involved have reached the appropriate stage of development (Stroand 1983). The process of bowel training during a child's development may have profound effects on bowel habits later in life.

During enforced delay in expulsion or when the defaecation reflex is ignored, the desire to defaecate wanes. The rectum can accommodate a distension of up to 400 ml, whilst still maintaining a low rectal pressure, and retrograde movement can propel the faeces back into the sigmoid colon. However, absorption of fluid and electrolytes continues so that retention of faeces leads to drier, harder stools that are difficult and painful to expel. Chronic delaying of the act of defaecation and tolerance of faeces in the rectum can be associated with constipation.

Constipation

Constipation is a subjective and variable symptom, not an actual disease process. There is no universally accepted definition, which may cause confusion and variation in the way it is managed. The term constipation may relate to slowness or infrequency of bowel movements and/or to the state of the stool. A popular definition, presumably because it relates to several factors, is 'infrequent, irregular passage of hard faeces with difficulty and occasional pain' (Lack & Twycross 1986).

In order to define constipation, it is crucial to identify what is 'normal defaecation' and the variations within this normal range. Epidemiology suggests that 95% of people in the USA and UK pass three stools per week (Bartolo & Wexner 1995). The normal range is between three times a day to three times a week (Roberts 1987). In general, constipation can be considered as a deviation from an individual's normal pattern, in the presence of additional factors such as straining and discomfort.

NURSING ASSESSMENT OF CONSTIPATION

Nursing assessment of those with actual or potential risk of constipation provides the foundation for individualised nursing management. The initial assessment should be updated as the individual's condition or treament changes.

Assessment of individuals should encompass a spectrum of 'biopsychosocial' factors. These are intricately linked and influence each other. The psychological aspects affecting constipation are complex, particularly as the subject is often perceived as taboo. Assessment should ideally occur within a private, non-threatening atmosphere. Questions should be posed using words acceptable to, and understood by, the patient. The questions outlined

---

Box 2.1 Suggested questions for the assessment of bowel function (adapted from Norton 1991)

- Patient's usual term for defaecation?
- Usual frequency of bowel action?
- Usual consistency and nature of stool?
- Usual time of day of bowel action?
- Any associated habits/events?
- Do patients feel they have a normal healthy bowel habit?
- What do they understand about constipation?
- Do they always respond to the urge to have their bowels open?
- Do they strain?
- How long does it take for their bowels to open?
- Is there any pain or bleeding associated?
- Do they take or avoid any food for their bowels?
- What is their average daily fluid intake?
- What is their past and present use of laxatives, and with what success?
- What other medications do they take?
- What is their past medical history?
- What is their present medical situation?
- Have they any problems or changes in their environment, lifestyle, mobility or mood?
- Have they experienced any recent changes in bowel habit or new problems?

in Box 2.1 can be used to gain valuable information. However, assessment should include more than a collection of facts regarding bowel function; it can also provide a comprehensive picture of the patient's beliefs, fears, misconceptions and deficits in knowledge which may need to be addressed. Assessment may highlight socio-economic factors that influence a patient's bowel habit, such as environment, traditional use of laxatives and perceived normal social behaviour.

Assessment of bowel habit should be undertaken for all individuals admitted with gastroenterological problems. Established usual habits must be considered in order to anticipate and resolve potential or actual problems. Potential problems are the use of drug treatments or surgical intervention that may have constipating effects. Throughout the process of assesment, the nurse has an opportunity to increase a patient's awareness of the need to maintain or achieve a normal healthy bowel function.

The epidemiological study of constipation has yielded some interesting variables relating to age, gender and socio-economic class. However, studies only give a general overview, as they tend to have discrepancies in their definition of constipation and rarely compare primary and secondary causes.

Age has a strong influence on the prevalence of constipation and the subsequent frequency of visits to a doctor for the symptom. Constipation appears to increase after the age of 45 years, with an exponential rise after the age of 65. This tends not to be related to an increased transit time, but to an increased difficulty in passing faeces, with discomfort and straining being the main complaint. The rise in the incidence of constipation is considered multifactorial, but diet is the most important factor in the elderly, as the amount of food, and especially fibre decreases. Anorectal disorders, which are more common in the elderly population, are also important.

Women experience constipation during pregnancy and the puerperium, as the hormones progesterone and prostaglandin slow bowel peristalsis, as does the gravid uterus.

Socio-economic correlations to the prevalence of constipation have demonstrated that lower social classes, as determined by income, education level and occupation, report constipation more frequently. Differences cannot be attributed to a single factor, but it is thought likely that a low threshold to gain medical attention, poor diet and lifestyle factors all influence the likelihood of the symptom (Bartolo & Wexner 1995).

INVESTIGATIONS INTO BOWEL FUNCTION

The causes of constipation may be described in two broad categories. Primary constipation has its origin in a variety of factors such as inadequate diet, poor fluid intake, lack of exercise, environmental changes, emotional disturbances and ignoring the urge to defaecate. Secondary constipation has its origins in a disease process or surgical and/or medical regimes. Examples are conditions such as painful anorectal disease, e.g. fissures, megacolon, diverticular disease, colonic tumours, hypercalcaemia or intake of iron supplements.

Constipation of unknown cause requires investigation before treatment is instigated. The nurse has a key role in assessing bowel function, as outlined previously. When secondary constipation is suspected, the nurse can provide invaluable support and information regarding the process of medical investigation. This includes ensuring the patient can give informed consent for the investigation and that they are fully prepared for the nature and duration of the invasive procedure. Nurses may provide information verbally or with the use of printed leaflets.

Throughout the investigative procedures, the nurse should ensure that the patient is comfortable and relaxed, with pain relief offered where appropriate. The embarrassment suffered during investigations can be minimised by maintaining dignity where possible. Reassurance can be given that involuntary passing of faeces is unlikely during internal investigations.

The digital rectal examination is performed to ascertain the presence, type and volume of faeces in the rectum, with the glove being inspected for blood and mucus. The examination may reveal carcinomas, as many occur in the lowest 12 cm of the large bowel, or defective sphincter control. Proctoscopy and rigid sigmoidoscopy provide visualisation of the mucosa up to 60 cm from the anal margin; this may reveal haemorrhoids, anal fissures, rectal carcinomas or diverticulitis, all of which can lead to constipating symptoms.

Colonoscopy enables inspection of the entire large bowel including the caecum; it requires bowel preparation to facilitate visualisation and is usually performed with sedation. Colonoscopy may reveal diverticular disease, or the presence of colonic polyps, tumour or ulceration.

Double contrast Barium enema (barium and gas) may distinguish gross abnormalities by demonstrating size, length and outline of the lumen of the colon, thus indicating the presence of megacolon, megarectum, volvulus, intussusception and tumours. The Guaiac test detects the presence of occult or 'hidden' blood in the faeces, a possible indication of colorectal cancer. The value of this test, however, is questionable, as it yields a high rate of false positives and negatives.

The patient may have specific investigations to exclude endocrine and metabolic causes of constipation. Constipation is a characteristic feature of hypothyriodism and is also seen in hypercalcaemia (Fig. 2.2).

NURSING MANAGEMENT OF PRIMARY CONSTIPATION

Primary constipation may be managed by focusing on the most natural means of promoting a healthy bowel action which the individual can maintain. When investigations have excluded secondary causes of constipation, information obtained from nursing assessment management should be directed towards:

- achieving the appropriate dietary intake of fibre and the appropriate type and volume of fluids
- improving bowel habit by responding to the urge to defaecate as soon as possible
- promotion of healthy posture of defaecation
- achievement of fitness through exercise to assist healthy bowel action
- minimising psychological factors that may hinder regular bowel actions
- promoting environmental factors that assist easy, undisturbed toileting

- providing information (and ensuring it is understood) regarding the maintenance of healthy bowel habits, appropriate to individual needs.

Bowel habits

Individuals' normal bowel habit is shaped by preference, lifestyle and their usual environment. The perception of what is a 'normal' bowel habit varies greatly. A detailed nursing assessment will pinpoint an unusual bowel habit that may be detrimental to healthy regular bowel action and may be the major predisposing factor leading to simple constipation.

Perhaps one of the simplest and healthiest approaches to bowel habit is to respond to the 'urge to defaecate'. This urge is often initiated by the process of eating, especially after a period of fasting, for example at breakfast after a night's sleep. The stimulus provokes a 'gastrocolic reflex', giving rise to a massive colonic contraction. On assessment, it may be discovered that individuals are ignoring this reflex, as they may be rushing to work or they may feel it is inappropriate or even too bothersome to go at that time. Persistent failure to respond promptly to the urge to defaecate can give rise to primary constipation. The nurse should explain how important it is to respond to the reflex, and advise individuals to set aside undisturbed time to have a bowel movement when the reflex occurs.

The process of hospitalisation may disturb individuals' 'normal' bowel habits, as they may have patterns based around activities difficult to mimic in hospital, e.g. after a cigarette, reading the paper or walking the dog. The nurse needs to be sensitive to these changes, and should demonstrate creativity to accommodate individuals' habits. Reassurance must be given to patients if their normal bowel action is disturbed, and appropriate measures taken to correct the problem.

The nurse can ensure that individuals are not deterred from healthy bowel habits due to environmental factors. Simple issues are important, such as determining whether a patient is aware of the location of the toilet and can gain easy access to it. Mobility and visual acuity should be assessed, so that provisions can be made to enable independent and safe access to a toilet. Large toilet signs, manageable locks, lights and the provision of handrails, call buttons and elevated toilet seats may all ease the process.

The patient may ignore the urge to defaecate due to embarrassment about requiring assistance with the removal of clothing, positioning and attending to hygiene needs. Reassurance and understanding demonstrated by nursing staff can reduce the embarrassment felt, and provision should be made to promote independence where possible.

Perhaps the most significant environmental factor that may deter healthy bowel habits is the toilet facility itself. Toilets which are dirty, odorous, cold, dimly lit or surrounded by unemptied bed pans may be considered highly constipating!

If a patient is unable to walk or be wheelchaired to a toilet cubicle then the use of a commode by the bedside may be unavoidable. However, the thought or act of defaecation whilst in the same room as others can cause extreme distress and embarrassment. The psychological impact should not be trivialised, and all measures should be taken to ensure maximum privacy. Dignity can be maintained by providing curtains around the bedside and by the unobtrusive use of a scented spray to minimise odours. Noises may also cause severe embarrassment, which can be minimised by the subtle use of radio or television as appropriate.

Patients may be extremely reluctant to request a commode in front of visiting friends and family. A diplomatic nurse would ask visitors to wait in a nearby day room or corridor, rather than outside the curtains and within earshot. The commode can then be provided and removed unobtrusively, and visitors called when it is appropriate to return. Some patients prefer a nurse to 'stand guard' while they are on the commode; this may provide reassurance and safeguard against unwary visitors or the uninvited ward round!

Overall, the individual who is hospitalised often has restricted freedom to continue a normal bowel habit. The nurse's assessment and care can enable normal habits to continue, whilst maintaining the patient's dignity and independence. Asking patients to wait or to go at a more convenient time is unacceptable. Toileting is a very basic aspect of nursing care, but done with respect and in a considered manner, it can have a profound influence on an individual's sense of well-being.

Posture and exercise

The correct posture for defaecation is considered important in promoting a good bowel habit. Crouching is considered anatomically to be the best position, although this is unfamiliar to most in the Western world. In the developed world, a more upright posture is usual, however a 'crouch-like' posture may be enhanced by flexing the patient's thigh and pelvis by the use of a footstool while sitting on the toilet.

Research has demonstrated that the posture whilst sitting on a bed pan can cause extreme straining during the process of defaecation. Bed pans are known to cause the greatest change in bowel habits for hospital in-patients, as compared with use of the commode and hospital toilets (Clark & Hodley 1979). If their use is unavoidable, the patient should be supported by pillows, so as to achieve the optimum upright position.

The use of straining to assist the passage of faeces produces a natural 'Valsalva' manoeuvre, which has inherent dangers. Although extremely rare, straining may give rise to serious complications, such as exacerbating existing cardiac disease or rupturing aneurysms. The movement may also dislodge clots, causing thromboembolic problems and resulting in cerebral or pulmonary emboli. Thirdly, the action of straining decreases respiratory function which may exacerbate a period of hypoxia. Less seriously, but nevertheless troublesome, straining can lead to and exacerbate the condition of haemorrhoids. The nurse needs to explain fully the serious risks involved in the simple process of straining and reassure the patient that measures can be taken to avoid straining.

Exercise is thought to prevent constipation and promote healthy bowel habits, because of its specific effect on gastrointestinal motility and its more general effect on muscle tone. Research to validate this is lacking. However, it seems that those who have chronic disabilities, impaired muscular function or a sedentary lifestyle are often prone to constipation. During defaecation, there is normally a contraction of abdominal and pelvic muscles; specifically exercising these muscles may enhance the treatment of primary constipation.

Psychological factors

The psychosocial aspects of bowel habits are influenced by a multitude of factors. Nurses may benefit from exploring an individual's perception of what is normal and assessing their attitude to constipation. Areas of relevance may include their memory of bowel training, cultural influences and environmental factors, all of which may have shaped and influenced their perception of what constitutes a normal bowel habit.

Constipation is a multifaceted disorder, with psychological factors both contributing to the cause of the dysfunction and resulting from it. Psychological factors contributing to the cause may be chronic: ignoring the urge to defaecate, abnormal eating patterns, extreme laxative abuse and living an unhealthy lifestyle. The psychological impact of disruption and discomfort caused by constipation may in turn lead to changes in personality and lifestyle, which may further exacerbate the problem. Individuals who are chronically constipated may change their eating behaviour, lessen their physical activity, and become depressed and socially withdrawn.

Chronic constipation has been linked to the development of paradoxical puborectalis contraction (PPC). This condition occurs when the puborectalis muscles and the external anal sphincter muscles contract during attempts to defaecate, thus obstructing the intent to open the bowels. This dysfunction of normal muscles is possibly linked to an abnormal learning process rather than to the persistence of an abnormal spasm (Bartolo & Wexner 1995). This contraction can be the cause of proctalgia fugax, a fleeting but severely intense pain in the rectum.

Once pelvic floor dysfunction has been identified as the cause of constipation (by manometric and electromyographic evaluation), this so-called 'outlet obstruction' may be modifiable by behavioural techniques.

Biofeedback is a learning strategy derived from psychological learning theory. Its theoretical basis is 'operant conditioning' or learning through reinforcement. For example, using external electrode pads placed around the anal sphincter muscle, the patient will receive visual feedback in the form of electromyorgraphic traces. A water-filled balloon is placed in the rectum to simulate stool. When asked to push the balloon out (simulate defaecation), the patient will be able to see the trace on the screen from the electrodes, which will give them information about whether or not they are relaxing the anal sphincter. Biofeedback is increasingly becoming the treatment of choice for many sufferers of constipation (Enck 1993).

Chronic constipation has been linked to so-called reflex signs such as headache, fatigue and vertigo. However, theories of auto-intoxication by the absorption of colonic toxins have not been proved. These sensations may be attributed to other symptoms such as dehydration (Wright 1974).

The anticipation of pain and discomfort may provoke an individual to avoid a bowel action and lead to worsening muscle tension and the development of PPC. Pain that is precipitated by the defaecation process, such as that caused by anal fissures, thrombosed haemorrhoids, injury or severe straining, may be avoided by the appropriate use of non-constipating analgesia and laxatives.

The psychology of bowel habits is complex and deep-seated. Psychologists often relate infant bowel training to adult habits. The mother's habits are thought to affect a child's attitude towards bowel function and to influence certain personality traits. It has been suggested that having an over-anxious mother can result in the toilet situation and training set-up assuming great proportions in the child's impressionable mind. Hence, later in adult life, the onset of stress or emotional disturbance may quickly lead to a breakdown in normal healthy bowel habit. Similarly, an extreme emphasis on bowel regularity as a child may later result in an adult obsession, leading to overuse of laxatives to ensure daily defaecation.

The effects of anxiety may predispose individuals towards constipation, although the exact effects of mood and attitude are difficult to establish clinically.

Patients with psychiatric problems can present with many bowel-related manifestations, including constipation. Depression leads to a disturbance of neurotransmitters that may alter bowel function and appetite. Some psychotropic drugs, such as the tricyclic antidepressants, may also exacerbate the condition.

Anorexia nervosa involves a poor dietary intake, lowered basal metabolic rate and emotional disturbances related to distorted body image. The physical consequences include constipation. Dementia involves the progressive generalised failure of higher cerebral function and can lead to apathy and inability to respond to the urge to defaecate, resulting in chronic constipation. Constipation may increase confusion in the elderly, although research in this area is scanty.

Dehydration

Insufficient fluid intake is a common contributing factor to the symptom of constipation. In healthy people, the volume and composition of body fluids are held remarkably constant; however, in disease this balance may be deranged as a result of extrarenal factors, e.g. vomiting, endocrine disturbances or intrinsic renal disease. Clinically, these imbalances should be addressed, by ensuring appropriate fluid replacement therapy with fluid balance assessment.

Most commonly, reduced fluid intake occurs as a consequence of reduced access to fluids and a diminished thirst mechanism in the hospitalised, elderly patient. The elderly may also be reluctant to take fluids due to a confused state or fear of exacerbating urinary incontinence (Murray 1992). Nurses can be proactive in ensuring that individuals are encouraged to have an intake of non-diuretic fluids up to 2–2.5 L/24 h; this may lessen the likelihood of constipation.

The common belief that drinking coffee has a laxative effect was researched by Brown et al (1990). Results from a questionnaire supported by manometric studies demonstrated that both caffeinated and decaffeinated coffee increased colonic motility. The studies showed that the response was not induced by temperature or volume, since hot water did not have a similar effect. The results are thought to show that coffee induces a strong 'gastrocolic effect', to be mediated by gastrointestinal hormones.

Modern diet and disease

Constipation may be regarded as endemic in developed societies. One hundred years ago, symptoms of constipation were uncommon in the West, as they are still in undeveloped rural communities.

Throughout evolution, humans as hunter-gatherers subsisted on a staple diet of vegetables, fruits, grain and legumes, with small amounts of meat and fish. The human gastrointestinal and metabolic systems are thus adapted to this high fibre diet. Since the Industrial Revolution, the Western diet has changed in response to convenience, fashion, affluence and food-refining technology. Overall, there has been a steady decline in the consumption of fibre and a corresponding increase in the consumption of refined carbohydrates, protein and saturated fats, with higher calorific values. Figures demonstrate an average value of 20 g fibre consumed per day in a Western diet, where constipation is prevalent. By contrast, rural dwellers in the developing world, with a diet similar to that of the hunter-gatherers, eat 100 g fibre per day.

Dietary fibre resists enzyme degradation and enters the colon, where it substantially increases faecal 'bulk' or volume. With soft, bulky stools, the colon is assisted in maintaining a larger lumen diameter, and consequently has a lower intraluminal pressure. A refined diet gives reduced bulk and smaller, harder stools; these require higher colonic pressures, because strong contractions are needed for propulsion. Overall, peristalsis is less effective, the hard stool increases friction and the smaller bulk may increase the concentration of potential carcinogens. The gastrointestinal transit time is decreased by the presence of fibre; hence, those in the developing world have an average transit time of $1\frac{1}{2}$ days, while those in the developed world have an average of 3 days. The shorter the transit time through the colon, the less opportunity there is for the absorption of water, giving rise to softer, wetter stools which can be easily evacuated.

Dietary fibre

The consumption of dietary fibre, coupled with adequate fluid intake, is the foundation of the prevention and treatment of constipation.

The definition of dietary fibre can be rather vague and misleading; variations include plant cellulose, unavailable carbohydrate, roughage and bulk. However, dietary fibre is not rough, nor is it an inert filler. Perhaps a more suitable definition is as follows: fibre is a general term for a widely diverse group of complex, non-starch carbohydrates of differing chemical structure and physical properties, which are not digestible by human intestinal enzymes (Taylor 1990).

Sufficient dietary fibre can maintain a healthy bacterial flora; the microbial mass and gases produced by their activity add bulk to the faeces. A high intake of dietary fibre can be an essential part of the management of many bowel conditions and the prevention of others. The substantial increase in a daily fibre diet can prevent and relieve constipation in almost all patients.

The challenge to the nurse is to make the introduction of fibre into an individual's normal dietary intake an effective and tolerable change. Firstly, the nurse/patient relationship should be a partnership whereby the patient believes and understands the nurse's information and practical advice. The nurse should empower patients to come to decisions regarding changes in diet and, where appropriate, utilise dieticians and doctors for information and additional support. A fundamental aspect of changing dietary habits is the inclusion and cooperation of friends, family and carers in assisting with compliance and providing encouragement.

Dietary fibre should include a wide variety of different fibres with differing properties. This is preferable to a refined diet supplemented with bran (see Box 2.2). The introduction of fibre to a diet should be gradual, over weeks or even months, and intake should be adjusted to the softness of the stool. The gradual intake may lessen the likelihood of secondary effects such as bloating, abdominal cramps and flatulence. Many of these unpleasant side-effects reduce with time, probably due to an alteration in colonic microflora (Cummings 1993).

Individuals' compliance with increasing fibre intake is often poor, especially in the elderly population where dietary habits are well established. Compliance may be affected by the fact that refined foods are often highly palatable in comparison to the more 'acquired' taste of high fibre foods. Advice should be given and appropriate literature supplied regarding tasty, desirable high fibre meals and snacks. The elderly may need advice regarding good dentition, as high fibre foods often demand more chewing. Compliance with increased fibre consumption may be sustained if its other virtues are explained fully, as outlined in Box 2.3.

Bulk forming drugs

Bulk forming drugs act in a similar fashion to dietary fibre, bulking faeces and reducing transit time. Preparations include methylcellulose (Celevac),

---

Box 2.2 High fibre foods

- Whole grain and bran enriched breakfast cereals, e.g. All Bran (not cornflakes, puffed rice, etc.)
- Unpeeled fruit and vegetables (although low in fibre compared with grains and pulses)
- Wholemeal bread (not white or 'brown')
- Whole wheat products, e.g. pasta
- Whole grains, e.g. brown rice, sweetcorn
- Pulses, e.g. kidney beans, lentils
- Nuts
- Dried fruit (raisins, apricots, prunes, etc.).

Box 2.3 Properties of dietary fibre

1. Decreases gastrointestinal transit time – reduces duration of contact between stool and bowel mucosa, and therefore potential contact of carcinogens, predisposing to rectal cancer
2. Reduces intraluminal pressure – reduces straining and subsequent conditions such as haemorroids and rectal prolapse
3. Reduces refined carbohydrate intake – fibre may reduce the incidence of maturity onset diabetes, as its presence reduces the opportunity for prolonged sugar absorption, and reduces the demand on B-cells in the islets of Langerhans to produce insulin
4. Reduces absorption of dietary fat – fibre may decrease fat absorption and blood lipid levels by its binding capacity and its effect on decreased transit time

---

sterculia (Normocol) and ispaghula husk (Fybogel, Regulan) which are all available as commercial non-prescription medications. These drugs must be taken with appropriate fluid intake 2–3 L/day non-diuretic fluids). The preparations swell in contact with liquid, and therefore should be taken with plenty of water. Patients should be advised not to take preparations before going to bed, so as to reduce the risk of obstructive symptoms. Potentially harmful effects may include exacerbation of constipation if inadequate fluid is taken, malabsorption of minerals, calcium, iron and fat-soluble vitamins, and reduced bioavailability of some drugs.

These preparations may reduce appetite and result in a lowered food intake, giving the potential for malnutrition. Bulk forming drugs may only take effect after several days, which the patient should be made aware of, and should be continued on a regular basis. The main contraindications to their use are in suspected subacute obstruction (e.g. Crohn's disease or carcinoma) and in neurological disease (paralysis).

Laxative management of constipation

Laxatives are medicines which promote a bowel action. Various synonyms are used to describe them: purgatures, (purifying) aperients, (opening) evacuents and cathartics. Laxative consumption is a widespread phenomenon and has been described as the commonest type of drug abuse in the Western world. Reasons for taking these over-the-counter medicines are steeped in misconceptions and enduring myths. Primarily, the belief in and desire to have a daily bowel action continues, and therefore laxatives are taken to ensure this happens and to 'prevent' constipation. Research has found that the bowel-conscious population tends to include the young and the elderly, and is predominantly female.

With the traditional and ritualistic practices associated with the use of unprescribed laxatives, nurses along with GPs and pharmacists have a vital role to play, through advice and education, in breaking the cycle of laxative dependence.

MANAGEMENT OF SECONDARY CONSTIPATION

Primary constipation can usually be successfully managed by correcting causative factors such as poor fibre intake, low fluid intake, inactivity, poor posture and ignoring call to stool, as described previously. The use of appropriate laxatives may be necessary in the initial stage. However, patients with certain gastroenterological conditions, surgery, disease states or drug regimes may require long-term use of laxative therapy for secondary constipation.

Common gastroenterological conditions which can present with secondary constipation are described below.

Diverticular disease occurs as a result of chronic constipation due to years of a low fibre diet, causing hypertrophy of the colonic muscle wall. The increased intraluminal pressures result in pockets of mucosa herniating through natural areas of weakness. The presence of the diverticula is often asymptomatic. Occasionally (5% of cases), inflammation can lead to diverticulitis, pericolic abscess, intraperitoneal perforation, fistula formation, bowel strictures and adhesions. Diverticula are so common in older patients that they are considered normal.

Chronic grumbling diverticular pain is the most common manifestation. For many patients, symptoms may be relieved by a high fibre diet and bulking agents, and these may correct the chronic constipation.

Irritable bowel syndrome is a common condition which has characteristic symptoms of cramping abdominal pain, bloating and erratic bowel habit. Colonic motility is deranged, giving rise to high intraluminal pressures and segmenting non-propulsive contractions. Faeces become dehydrated and fragmented, giving rise to constipation associated with hard 'pellet-like' stools. Treatment again involves adequate fibre diet, bulking agents and, where necessary, antispasmodic drugs (see discussion on p. 51).

Colonic pseudobstruction, which occurs in patients who have long-standing constipation or chronic laxative abuse, is not uncommon in the elderly and mentally handicapped. The colon develops into a capacious, elongated and relatively atonic loop, which can become twisted producing a closed loop obstruction known as a sigmoid volvulus.

Haemorrhoids, commonly known as piles, are displaced anal cushions. The vascular cushions help seal the upper anal canal and contribute to continence. They are displaced by straining to pass small, hard, constipated stools. Increased intra-abdominal pressure inhibits venous return and causes the venous cushions to become engorged. Persistent straining can cause the pelvic floor to sag causing prolapse. Overall, episodes of constipation are the precipitating factor in haemorrhoids, which can be corrected by the introduction of a high fibre diet and bulking agents. Patients need to be advised not to spend great lengths of time on the toilet, reading for example. This habit can easily lead to unnecessary straining at the end of defaecation, when the haemorrhoids or rectal prolapse can actually feel like the incomplete evacuation of faeces.

An anal fissure is a split in the mucosa and skin of the anal canal, usually caused by the passage of a large constipated stool. The fissure causes sphincter spasm which can prevent healing. Conservative treatment involves the use of anaesthetic gel and measures to resolve passing constipated stool.

Solitary rectal ulcers occur on the anterior wall of the rectum and arise as a result of repeated mucosal trauma. This happens characteristically with straining on hard constipated stool, or using fingers or objects to aid defaecation (Carlson et al 1993).

Slow transit constipation is a gross form of constipation, sometimes referred to as colonic inertia. The condition occurs in individuals who are otherwise in good health, predominantly young women who present with abdominal cramps and distension, with passage of stools as infrequent as every 2–4 weeks. The condition can be difficult to treat, as it is thought to be due to a muscular disorder of the colon. Treatment requires lifelong use of osmotic laxatives. Stimulant laxatives should be avoided except in a crisis, since regular use exacerbates the condition. Large volumes of osmotic laxatives (60–120 ml lactulose daily) may be needed.

The term megacolon is used to describe a number of conditions in which the colon is dilated. All young patients with megacolon need to have Hirshsprung's disease excluded. This congenital abnormality usually presents in the first years of life, due to an aganglionic segment of the rectum causing constipation and subacute obstruction. The disease can be confined to the distal segment of the rectum and can be missed in childhood. A fullthickness rectal biopsy, using special stains for ganglion cells in the submucosal plexus, should be performed for adult patients with megacolon. The disease may be treated surgically by resection of the aganglionic segment.

Endocrine disturbances

Secondary constipation as a result of endocrine disturbances may be treated by controlling the endocrine condition, e.g. thyroxine for hypothyroidism.

Pharmacological management

In severe constipation, immediate treatment often requires the temporary use of laxatives, followed by long-term prophylactic measures. Oral laxatives of any kind are contraindicated if there is any suggestion of bowel obstruction.

The prescription of laxatives should be made with an informed regard for their actions and side-effects, while also bearing in mind type and extent of constipation. Patients should be included in the management programme, and their needs listened to, with advice regarding laxative use made explicit.

Local laxative measures

Lubricant glycerine suppositories. These act by virtue of a mildly irritant action, which has a softening effect on hard dry faeces. The suppository needs to be inserted directly into the faeces, having been moistened with water.

Stimulant suppository (e.g. bisacodyl) This acts by increasing rectal motility through its contact with the rectal mucous membrane; it acts within 20–60 min and may give rise to colicky pains.

Small phosphate and sodium citrate enemas (disposable or 'mini' enemas). These act by changing the pattern of water distribution in the faeces, which is particularly helpful when chronic constipation causes faecal soiling due to a loaded rectum.

Stool softening arachis oil enemas. These act by penetrating faeces, increasing the bulk and softness of stools. The enema works most effectively when warmed and retained for as long as possible (Clark 1988).

Large volume soap and water enemas. The use of high volume enemas are now contraindicated due to the serious risk of causing circulatory overload and colonic perforation, water intoxication, mucosal necrosis and hyperkalaemia. The administration of large amounts of fluid may cause breakdown of an anastomosis, perforation or haemorrhage, especially to an ulcerated or inflamed bowel. However, enemas have been an historic part of health culture and their use as a cleansing agent has been in vogue at times. Patients should be warned of the inherent dangers associated with their use.

Oral laxative agents

Bulk forming laxatives (see p. 38).

Stimulant/irritant laxatives (e.g. senna, bisacodyl, danthron). The active component of these drugs is produced by their metabolism by colonic bacteria. The drug stimulates submucosal nerve plexuses, increasing motility and secretion of water and electrolytes into the colon.

The chronic use of stimulant laxatives may lead to the development of 'melanosis coli'. This is a hyperpigmentation of the colonic mucosa, which has a minimal physiological effect, but is a marker of laxative abuse. However, some patients develop an atonic colon due to chronic laxative abuse over 20–40 years, and may require stimulant laxatives in infrequent minimal dosages, in order to ensure a bowel action. Generally, the use of laxatives should be considered a short-/medium-term treatment, in addition to long-term prophylactic measures, e.g. dietary fibre and increased fluid intake to promote a normal healthy bowel action.

Danthron is principally used as co-danthramer and co-danthrusate; however, its use is limited due to recent research which has suggested a potential carcinogenic risk. Nevertheless, its use continues in terminally ill patients with drug-induced constipation, and in elderly care.

Faecal softeners and lubricants (e.g. liquid paraffin, docusate sodium). These act by coating the outside of faeces and inhibiting fluid absorption. Liquid paraffin should not be taken at bedtime, so as to minimise the risk of nocturnal reflux and aspiration which can give rise to lipoid pneumonia. Docusate sodium (Dioctyl) acts both as a stimulant and as a softening agent.

Osmotic laxatives (e.g. lactulose, magnesium hydroxide (milk of magnesia) and magnesium sulphate (Epsom salts)). Many magnesium-based osmotic laxatives are not available on the NHS. They are useful when rapid bowel evacuation is required, but are strongly contraindicated for patients with renal and/or hepatic impairment.

Non-absorbable sugars such as lactulose act by their osmotic effect. Their presence in the bowel draws fluid into the lumen, thus ensuring moist, soft faeces. Lactulose is a very acceptable, effective laxative. Its sweetness may be

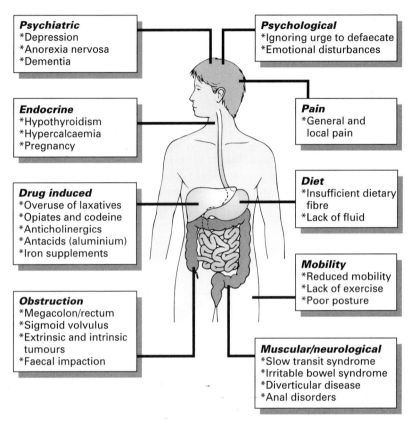

Fig 2.2 Causes of constipation.

diluted with fruit juice, and it is suitable for those with diabetes mellitus. Its action may occur 3 hours after administration or up to 48 hours later.

Strong laxative for single-dose use, such as in bowel preparation or very stubborn constipation (e.g. sodium picosulphate – Picolax). These stimulant laxatives are used only for bowel preparation or extremely resistant constipation. They must be used with extreme caution, as they can precipitate abdominal cramps, fluid loss and hypokalaemia. Their laxative effect occurs within 3 hours of the first dose.

Non-prescription laxatives (e.g. rhubarb extract, aloes, jalap). These should all be advised against, due to their unpredictable purgative actions.

Faecal impaction
Chronic constipation can result in the impaction of faeces in the rectum, which become harder and drier with continued absorption of fluid. Problems arise when there is a hard core of faeces which becomes too large to pass

through the anus. The rectum overdistends and accommodates the mass. Mucus production and bacterial action cause liquefaction of constipated faeces; this leaks around the mass and escapes as 'spurious', or overflow, diarrhoea. Patients often lack awareness or control of the diarrhoea, which results in a constant leakage of offensive liquid stool.

Management

Initial treatment is to empty the rectum until the faecal mass is cleared. This is performed with daily suppositories, enemas or occasionally with manual removal using gentle finger manipulation. Some elderly patients have massive rectal impaction with soft faeces.

Long-term management is to keep the rectum empty by preventing recurrence of constipation. In elderly immobile patients prone to this condition, this may be best managed by regularly using appropriate laxatives at the minimal effective dose.

DIARRHOEA

Diarrhoea may be defined as the passing of increased amounts (>300 g/24 h) of loose stool. True diarrhoea is different from the frequent passage of small amounts of stool, which is commonly seen in functional bowel disease, e.g. irritable bowel syndrome, postvagotomy, and conditions such as hyperthyroidism (Clark 1990). This occurs as a result of hypermotility of the gastrointestinal tract and reduced contact time for fluid reabsorption, giving rise to loose stools of normal volume.

True diarrhoea may be classified according to duration (acute or chronic) or type (secretory, osmotic or mixed). The pathophysiology varies among these different classifications of diarrhoea (see Fig. 2.3).

Osmotic diarrhoea

Osmotic diarrhoea occurs when there are large quantities of 'hypertonic' substances in the gastrointestinal tract which exert an osmotic pressure and reduce reabsorption of water from the ileum and colon. Malabsorption syndromes are often chronic disorders which arise as a consequence of impaired digestion or absorption of food. Thus they can arise from lack of digestive enzymes (e.g. chronic pancreatic inflammation – pancreatitis) or due to small-intestinal villous atrophy in coeliac disease.

Malabsorbed nutrients may be fermented to organic acids by colonic bacteria, which promote salt and water secretion by the colon. Investigations into malabsorption syndromes, such as hydrogen breath tests, oral tolerance tests and jejunal brush border enzyme assays, reveal enzyme deficiencies and defects in assimilating nutrients. Sometimes patients can highlight associations with foodstuffs, e.g. association with milk ingestion and diarrhoea for those with lactose intolerance. With many patients, the association with the offending sugars is difficult to find. Diarrhoea may stop with avoidance of particular foodstuffs. Osmotic diarrhoea may be caused by ingestion of significant amounts of poorly absorbed substances, e.g. sorbitol, which is contained in many liquid medications, and osmotic laxatives such as magnesium

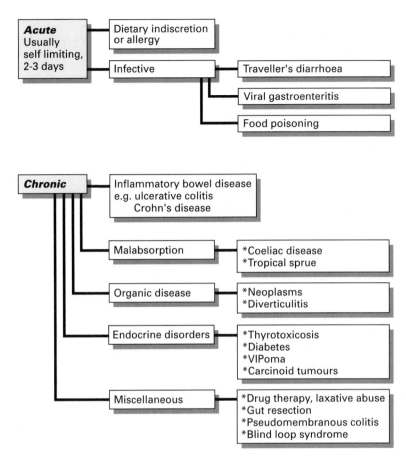

Fig 2.3   Causes of diarrhoea.

sulphate and lactulose. The diarrhoea ceases when the patient stops eating or the malabsorptive substance is discontinued. This is a simple but valuable distinguishing factor which occurs during a fast of 24–48 hours.

Secretory diarrhoea

With secretory diarrhoea, gastrointestinal cells exhibit abnormal ion transport, causing both secretion of fluid and electrolytes and decreased absorption. Secretory diarrhoea classically occurs with infection from a toxin-producing organism such as *Vibrio cholera* or *Escherichia coli*. These bacteria produce toxins that cause Cl^- secretion and inhibit Na^+ and Cl^- absorption, by their action on cell metabolism.

Certain rare disease states, such as carcinoid tumours (originating from serotonin-producing intestinal cells) and VIPomas (pancreatic tumours producing vasoactive intestinal peptides), cause severe intestinal secretion and watery diarrhoea. Ileal resection can lead to malabsorption of bile salts and

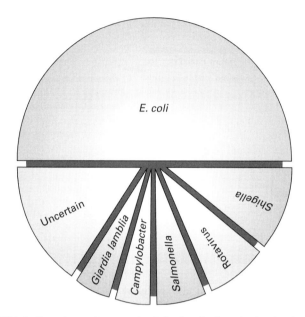

Fig 2.4   Distribution of organisms causing infective diarrhoea in the developed world.

fatty acids in the colon, which increase fluid secretion and give rise to diarrhoea.

In contrast to osmotic diarrhoea, secretory diarrhoea does not subside on fasting; in fact, nutrients are absorbed normally and glucose can enhance absorption of fluid and electrolytes. Secretory volumes can be very high (>2000 g/day).

Inflammatory diarrhoea

Diarrhoea occurs due to intestinal mucosal cell damage, causing increased permeability, with loss of fluid, electrolytes and blood. Inflammatory mediators provoke intestinal or colonic secretion. The damage also results in defective fluid absorption and increased intestinal motility. The commonest causes are infective conditions such as dysentery due to *Shigella* sp. and inflammatory conditions e.g. ulcerative colitis and Crohn's disease (see Chapter 4).

Diarrhoea induced by laxative abuse

This uncommon form of diarrhoea has been found predominantly in young women. Due to the great care individuals can take to conceal their habit, it is essential to eliminate this possible cause, before more extensive and expensive investigations are performed. Laxatives can be identified by chemical analysis of faeces or by colorimetric tests on urine. Patients may be hypokalaemic, or have indications of melanosis coli. Laxative abuse often occurs in cases of Bulimia nervosa, under the assumption that food can be flushed through the system unabsorbed. Management is often difficult, as the individual may deny laxative abuse. However, advice, reassurance and psychiatric support may be appropriate.

Pseudomembranous colitis

This antibiotic-associated diarrhoea is the commonest cause of hospital/medical institutional diarrhoea. The causative agent is *Clostridium difficile*, which selectively proliferates when the normal inhibitory microflora population is decreased, usually by a prescribed antibiotic. The clinical picture may be a mild attack of diarrhoea or profuse colitis. The condition of pseudomembranous colitis refers to a thick blanket of 'pseudomembrane', which forms on the mucosal surface after a period of severe inflammation. This membrane harbours the toxin-producing bacteria, causing worsening diarrhoea which may become chronic or relapsing. The bacteria and toxin can be identified by stool microscopy and culture. Treatment involves stopping current antibiotics and, if necessary, administering oral metronidazole or oral vancomycin. This condition should be considered in patients with diarrhoea following antibiotics, or in patients with an exacerbation of ulcerative colitis or renal failure.

Acute diarrhoea

Acute diarrhoea of sudden onset is very common, often short-lived and requires no investigation or treatment. This type of diarrhoea is seen after dietary indiscretions and abuse of alcohol. Infective diarrhoeas occur with a wide range of bacteria and viruses, the most common route of infection being ingestion. Infection of the gastrointestinal tract is known as enteritis. Routes of transmission are varied; the most common is the faecal–oral or hand-to-mouth spread, in which a breakdown in simple hygiene allows ingestion of contaminated faecal matter. Simple contamination of food or water by the same sources may occur. Food poisoning occurs with the production of toxins or due to multiplication of pathogens in food, sometimes surviving as spores during boiling, e.g. *Staphylococcus aureus*, *Bacillus cereus*, *Salmonella enteritidis*, *Clostridium botulinum*. The symptoms of bacterial food poisoning all involve diarrhoea and often vomiting, colitis and, in severe cases, systemic illness. Non-microbial toxins are found in shellfish, some spoiled fish and red kidney beans that have been partially cooked, giving rise to acute diarrhoea.

Travellers' diarrhoea occurs as individuals are exposed to unfamiliar pathogens, many whilst travelling from developed to developing countries. Most attacks last 2–3 days and are self-limiting (Fig. 2.4). However, recurring diarrhoea after an acute episode abroad may need to be investigated. Persistent infections can occur with *Giardia lamblia*, amoebiasis, *Campylobacter* sp., *Yersinia* sp. and *Shigella* sp. Physiological changes may occur as a result of an infective agent. For example, tropical sprue is diagnosed in the presence of malabsorption due to stunting of villi and histological changes. More commonly, diarrhoea may persist due to a postinfective irritable bowel syndrome, which may occur as a result of changes in normal colonic microflora (Turnberg 1987).

Miscellaneous types of diarrhoea

Drug-induced diarrhoea may occur as a result of drugs changing the bacterial flora, or having a direct toxic effect on the mucosa, e.g. antihypertensive drugs, diuretics, antacids or digoxin. Excessive alcohol consumption could also cause diarrhoea. In a number of systemic diseases, diarrhoea is a common feature and occasionally it may be the presenting and most prominent symptom, e.g. thyrotoxicosis, autonomic neuropathy in diabetes. Some chronic diarrhoea states have been attributed to nervous dispositions that affect colonic motility.

Stool samples need to be sent for culture and sensitivity tests that will detect bacterial growth and identify organisms, and for microscopy which can detect parasites and ova. Stool specimens can also be tested for the presence of laxatives, fat and blood.

Assessment may involve invasive medical investigations. Possible procedures include endoscopy for aspiration of intestinal contents and culture of bacterial overgrowth, and biopsies for coeliac sprue or Crohn's disease. Colonoscopy may detect inflammatory bowel disease, neoplasms or the presence of melanosis coli, indicating laxative abuse.

NURSING ASSESSMENT OF DIARRHOEA

The nursing assessment of patients wiht diarrhoea is vital for tailoring appropriate management and individualised care. Assessment needs to be continuously updated, as the condition can rapidly change. Useful questions to ask and areas to investigate are as follows:

- Patient's usual term for an episode of diarrhoea
- Usual frequency, time of day and nature of urgency
- Usual time spent having bowel actions
- Consistency of stool; presence of blood, fat, mucus
- Symptoms associated with diarrhoea, e.g. pain, fever, nausea, vomiting, fatigue, weight loss
- Have they any perianal problems?
- Ability to drink sufficient fluids
- Recent dietary changes, or correlation of diarrhoea to foodstuffs
- Normal medications, recent antibiotics or laxatives
- Effectiveness of antidiarrhoeal medication
- Family history of altered bowel habits
- Recent lifestyle changes, emotional disturbances or travel abroad
- How do they feel about the diarrhoea?

Assessment involves finding out about the stool characteristics and defaecation pattern, as well as the symptoms resulting from the diarrhoea.

A chart documenting the time, volume and nature of stool passed may provide useful information in the diagnosis of the cause. For example, large volume diarrhoea is characteristic of a disorder or disease of the small intestine or proximal colon. Other characteristics are lightly coloured, foul-smelling, watery stools with undigested food particles. Associated pain is usually intermittent, cramping and occurring in the periumbilical or right lower quadrant. Small volume diarrhoea is associated with the colon and rectum; stools are mushy with presence of mucus and/or blood. Urges to defaecate are frequent, are associated with aching pain in lower quadrants and rectal area and are often relieved by a bowel movement.

NURSING MANAGEMENT OF DIARRHOEA

After the cause of diarrhoea has been ascertained, nursing management should focus on:

- resolving the cause of diarrhoea
- re-establishing normal bowel function
- relieving symptoms, e.g. pain, nausea and vomiting, pyrexia
- maintaining comfort and hygiene
- minimising risk of complications, e.g. fluid and electrolyte imbalance
- reducing psychological distress
- providing information and education regarding condition.

Resolving the cause of diarrhoea must be tailored to the specific diagnosis and managed in conjunction with medical therapy.

Predominantly, the chronic diarrhoeas are managed with drug therapy, e.g. ulcerative colitis, Crohn's disease, or with specific dietary and fluid management, e.g. malabsorption syndromes. Acute diarrhoea is often short-lived and requires little treatment; management focuses on resolving symptoms and preventing complications.

The first line of nursing care is the prevention and/or correction of dehydration during an episode of diarrhoea. Assessment of dehydration can be made by establishing whether the patient has a dry mouth, dry mucous membranes or dry skin. The patient may report feelings of fatigue and dizziness. Signs of dehydration are a postural drop in diastolic blood pressure of >20 mmHg from normal levels, and a rise in pulse rate >20 beats per minute from the normal values. Clinical signs would demonstrate deranged serum urea and electrolyte levels, and a negative fluid balance.

The nurse records all fluid input and output regularly to determine the balance that prevails. A negative fluid balance demonstrates a net loss of fluid; insensible losses, such as sweating, of up to 1000 ml should be considered especially if the patient is pyrexial.

Fluid replacement may be achieved by simple measures. Nurses can encourage patients to take extra fluids, catering for their particular taste preferences. A full explanation should be given to patients and reassurance that drinking fluids will not worsen the diarrhoea, as this misconception is common.

Moderate dehydration may be corrected with the use of oral rehydration supplements. These have their effect on the basis that absorption of fluid and electrolytes is considerably enhanced by the addition of glucose. The solutions used in the UK are lower in sodium and higher in glucose than the WHO formulation. They are therefore only of benefit in mild to moderate diarrhoea, when the body's homeostatic mechanisms are functional, but would be suboptimal for correcting severe fluid losses and electrolyte imbalance as seen in the populations of developing countries (Carlson et al 1993). Solutions available are Dioralyte and Rehydrat, which enhance fluid and electrolyte absorption and replace the electrolyte deficiency.

The oral intake of fluids may be met with considerable reluctance. Nurses need to be creative and use ingenuity to make drinking less of an ordeal for the patient. Simple measures such as adding flavour, using ice and using the patient's own cup may all help. An essential aspect is ensuring that the patient is free from sensations such as nausea, by administering antiemetics, and is pain-free, by the appropriate use of analgesia. For patients who are reluctant or unable to take oral hydration, or for those who are seriously dehydrated, the administration of intravenous fluids is required. This must be prescribed to replenish deficits and to correct continuing losses, in order to restore normal fluid and electrolyte levels.

The symptomatic treatment of diarrhoea with medications has limitations. In acute diarrhoea, the antimotility drugs may be used as temporary measures, but may actually worsen infective diarrhoea by slowing the clearance of infective agents. Antimotility drugs available include codeine phosphate, co-phenotrope and loperamide.

Nursing management to promote comfort and maintain hygiene is a vital aspect of ensuring that the episode of diarrhoea is minimally traumatic. The nurse should ensure that the environment is appropriate for easy and rapid access to toilet facilities. Cleanliness of the environment, availability of washing facilities, clean linen and bedclothes are essential. The individual suffering from diarrhoea often feels intense embarrassment and may feel 'dirty', and may thus have a negative body image. All efforts must be made to facilitate privacy and to assist in attending to hygiene needs in a reassuring, respectful manner. Advice should be given regarding the potential or actual problem of soreness to the anal area and pruritis. After every bowel action, it is recommended to wash the anal area with a soft cloth or disposable wipe. Soap- and alcohol-based wipes should be discouraged as they may dry the skin. An emollient or protective paste such as Comfeel cream may offer local relief and protect the area.

The symptom of diarrhoea often occurs with episodes of cramping pain, and so the appropriate use of analgesia and evaluation of its effectiveness is an essential part of symptom relief. Diarrhoea is often associated with severe fatigue and sleep deprivation. The nurse can ensure that adequate rest periods are encouraged when visitors and other distractions are avoided.

Pyrexia may occur during infective diarrhoea. Relief may be provided by cold drinks, fans, cold compresses and regular administration of an antipyretic medication such as paracetomol. Antibiotics are not indicated for diarrhoea, except for the immunosuppressed patient or those with severe sepsis.

Nursing management of infective diarrhoea

Cases of acute diarrhoea must be considered potentially infectious until otherwise indicated. Precautions must be taken to minimise the risk of spread to others; advice may be sought from an infection control team if appropriate. Universal precautions involve the correct wearing and handling of protective gowns and gloves. Contaminated waste and utensils should be dealt with according to established policies. All excreta and vomit should be disposed of immediately. The patient may remain infectious even when signs and symptoms have subsided; the usual policy is for three negative stool results to be obtained before precautions are lifted. Ideally, the patient should be nursed in a side room and have access to their own designated toilet or commode.

Advice and reassurance should be given to family and friends, who should be encouraged not to be in direct contact with the patient. The elderly and the very young should be discouraged from visiting while the diarrhoea is still infective.

Psychological care

Central to all nursing care is the emphasis on the whole patient, not just the symptom. Diarrhoea, both acute and chronic, has a profound psychological and social impact on an individual. The loss of control and the self-disgust individuals may experience can lead to severe distress and, in some chronic situations, depression. Nurses can develop a therapeutic partnership with a patient by acknowledging the distress they are suffering and helping them to call on positive coping mechanisms. By discussing freely how they feel about the symptom, the effect it has on their body image and perceived social roles, the nurse can help patients verbalise their fears and anxieties. By giving time to demonstrate care and genuine concern for the individual, the nurse can foster a sense of self-worth and well-being for the patient.

Diarrhoea is a particularly taboo and antisocial symptom within our society. Individuals may experience intense social isolation from family and friends, thus increasing feelings of loneliness. Nurses may address this problem by acting as a catalyst to promote discussion, openness and understanding of the condition.

Those who suffer chronic diarrhoea symptoms require a great deal of support and education regarding the management of their condition. Individuals may find specific literature or access to support networks of great value.

IRRITABLE BOWEL SYNDROME

Irritable bowel syndrome (IBS) is one of the most common of the gastrointestinal disorders. It is also one of the least understood, because it is not a disease but a syndrome, made up of a number of conditions with similar manifestations.

IBS is a motor disorder characterised by a group of abdominal symptoms such as altered bowel habits, abdominal pain and the absence of any detectable organic disease. It is estimated that around 10% of the population suffer symptoms of IBS, but the actual prevalence of IBS is unknown. Data are scarce as it is not fatal and so does not appear as a cause of death on death certificates, and rarely requires admission to hospital. Nevertheless, the morbidity of IBS is significant, with statistics showing that in the past it ranked close to the common cold as a leading cause of absenteeism from work due to illness (Almy 1967).

More than twice as many women than men suffer from IBS in the Western world, although in India, more men than women present with IBS. These trends could reflect cultural care-seeking patterns, i.e. that men in developed countries do not refer to their GPs as often as women. Life experiences would also seem to contribute, as 44% of IBS patients report child sexual abuse.

Typical features include:

- age 20–40 years
- abdominal pain
- pelletty or ribbon-like stools
- obsessional personality
- bloating
- altered bowel habit
- duration >6 months
- unremarkable examination.

Less common features are:

- nausea
- dyspareunia
- depression (Travis et al 1993)
- pain in back, thigh or chest
- urinary frequency.

Symptoms appear to be markedly influenced by psychological factors such as stressful life situations. This, added to the absence of any detectable pathology, has contributed to the misconception that IBS is 'all in the mind'.

The causes of IBS are unclear, although gastroenteritis, prolonged courses of antibiotics, food sensitivities and abdominal surgery have all been proposed. There is a common association between IBS and minor gynaecological complaints, with many patients being referred from gynaecology clinics to the gastroenterology clinic.

Investigations

The aim of the gastroenterologist is to exclude organic disease using the minimum number of investigations. All patients will undergo urinalysis for protein or blood caused by a possible urinary tract infection. Blood tests will exclude many organic diseases with similar symptoms (ESR and full blood count). Stool culture will detect any infection. A rectal biopsy and sigmoidoscopy are always indicated. Other investigations are usually avoided unless there are unusual features.

Nursing contribution to the management of IBS

Once a diagnosis of IBS is made in the outpatients clinic, explanation of the symptoms is vital. The gastroenterologist is likely to provide this explanation, but the nurse, with sound knowledge of the facts, will be a valuable source of information and support to follow this up during this or subsequent visits.

The IBS sufferer is likely to have been told that the pain originates when small volume, hard stools cause the bowel muscle to contract harder than usual; that bowel spasm pain is like muscle cramp; that their bowel is more sensitive than normal and may be irritated by certain foods; and that the relation to stress is not an uncommon experience, e.g. pre-exam diarrhoea.

The likely pattern of the condition will be as follows:

- symptoms will continue for months or years, but will resolve eventually
- symptoms can be relieved but not always cured
- no risk of cancer
- reassure that there is something wrong, but it is not a disease; the bowel is more sensitive than normal (Travis et al 1993).

Diet
Many patients do have a specific food intolerance which can be identified by an exclusion diet (improvement of symptoms is possible in two-thirds of patients). Avoidance of these foods (e.g. onions, chocolate, lettuce) will bring relief. Reintroduction after 12 months is often possible, without relapse. The nurse in outpatients or in the community can play a valuable role in supporting the patient throughout the exclusion diet, reinforcing the value of it.

A high fibre diet can help when constipation is the predominant feature, although it can make flatulence or diarrhoea worse.

Drugs
Most patients prefer to manage without drugs, but they are used to treat symptoms when severe, e.g. antispasmodics for pain (mebeverine, but not when constipated); peppermint oil for bloating; osmotic laxative (e.g. lactulose) when constipated; loperamide (up to 12 daily) relieves frequency; metoclopramide for dyspepsia or nausea; amitriptylline (10–25 mg tds) to reduce gut motility when diarrhoea is persistent.

Stress management and alternative therapies of the patient's choice are found to be helpful by many. There is no uniform specific treatment, only suggestions of possibilities which the individual may find helpful.

Nursing intervention for this group of patients is almost entirely focused on enabling and supporting people to adapt their lives and use therapies to manage symptoms. As implied earlier, there is no panacea for IBS. There often appears to be a significant psychological component which may benefit tremendously from continuity of care. This may be either from a specialist gastroenterology nurse in the outpatient department, or even from seeing the same staff nurse at the clinic – one who is familiar, understands the syndrome and can listen and advise as indicated. Sufferers find that the trivialisation of their problems and talking to someone who is not listening are among the most trying aspects of coping with IBS. Nurses are in a position to set up trusting relationships with these people, to act as their advocate in situations where patients may feel their symptoms are being trivialised and to offer reassurance and enable self-management for the future.

REFERENCES

Almy T P 1967 Digestive disease as a national problem. II. A white paper by the
American Gastro. Association Gastroentology 53: 821
Bartolo D G C, Wexner S D 1995 Constipation: its etiology, evaluation and
management. Butterworth Heinmann, Philadelphia
Brown S R, Cann P A, Read N W 1990 Effect of coffee on distal colon function. GUT
31:450–453
Carlson G L, Wales S, Shaffer J L 1993 Drugs in the management of colorectal diseases.
In: Jones (ed), ABC of colorectal diseases. BMJ, London
Clark B 1988 Making sense of enemas. Nursing Times 84(30):40–41
Clark J M, Hodley L 1979 Research for nursing. A guide for the enquiring nurse. HM &
M Pub, Aylesbury, p 38–41
Cummings J H 1993 Nutritional management of bowel diseases. In: Garrow J S,
James W P T (eds) Human nutrition and dietetics, 9th edn. Churchill Livingstone,
Edinburgh
Enck P 1993 Digestive Diseases & Sciences 38(11):1953–1960
Lack S A, Twycross R G 1986 Control of alimentary symptoms in advanced cancer.
Churchill Livingstone, Edinburgh
Murray F E 1992 Constipation, an update on a common problem. Geriatric Medicine,
March:55–58
Norton C 1991 Eliminating In: Redfern S (ed) Nursing Elderly People 2nd edn.
Churchill Livingstone, Edinburgh
Roberts A 1987 Senior systems. Constipation. Nursing Times, Jan 14:37–38
Stroand F L 1983 A regulatory systems approach. Physiology, 2nd edn. Collier
McMillan, London
Taylor R 1990 Management of constipation. British Medical Journal 300:1064–1065
Travis S P L, Taylor R H, Misiewcz J J 1993 Gastroenterology, 2nd edn. Blackwell
Scientific, Oxford
Turnberg L A 1987 Clinical gastroenterology. Blackwell Scientific, Oxford
Wright D 1974 Bowel function in hospital patients. Royal College of Nursing, London,
ch 2, p 16–23

FURTHER READING

Castle C S 1987 Constipation: endemic in the elderly? Geriatric Medicine, Medical
Clinics of North America 73(6):1497–1503

Clark L M, Kumar J P 1990 Gastroenterology. In: Clinical medicine, 2nd edn. Ballière
Tindall, London

Lewin D 1976 Care of the constipated patient. Nursing Times, March 25:445–446

Molitor P 1985 Constipation. Nursing Mirror 160(19):18–21

Wright D 1984 Constipation two, the researcher's view. Nursing Times, May 30:65–67

Inflammatory bowel disease

Jill Hudson   Susan Goldthorpe

■ CONTENTS

OVERVIEW

In this chapter, two chronic non-specific inflammatory bowel disorders are discussed – ulcerative colitis and Crohn's disease. Initially, brief overviews of the disorders are given separately; perspectives on their respective treatments are then given and common aspects of patient care are considered. Figure 3.1 illustrates the relative position of the large and small bowel in the body.

Ulcerative colitis

Ulcerative colitis is an inflammatory disorder which affects the mucous membrane of the rectum and spreads proximally to involve part or all of the colon,

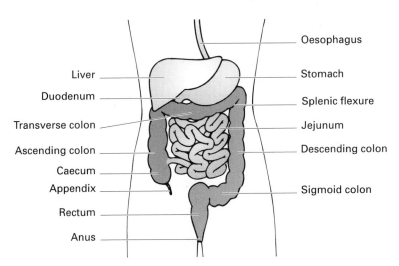

Fig 3.1 The position of the large and small bowel.

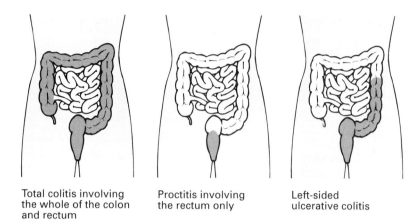

Total colitis involving the whole of the colon and rectum

Proctitis involving the rectum only

Left-sided ulcerative colitis

Fig 3.2 Areas affected in ulcerative colitis.

proctitis being more common than total colitis (see Fig. 3.2). It is characterised by remissions and relapses which can be months or years apart, although 10% of patients have continuous symptoms. The cure for ulcerative colitis is total colectomy, although many patients maintain remission from their symptoms with drug therapy.

Incidence and prevalence

The disease usually develops after puberty with a second peak in incidence between 55 and 70 years of age. It is most common in communities of Anglo-Saxon origin in the Western world. There appears to be a higher incidence in Jews than in other races. Preliminary studies suggest the incidence in Asian immigrants in the UK is similar to that in the indigenous population (Rhodes & Mayberry 1986).

About 80/100 000 of the population are affected and 10 new cases/100 000 are diagnosed each year:

- 15% of sufferers have a familial link to another sufferer
- it is twice as common in non-smokers than in smokers
- there are no recognised differences in gender (Travis et al 1993).

Pathology

Disease always arises in the rectal mucosa. It may spread back up (proximally) the colon, or the entire colon may be involved from the beginning, but the affected area is always continuous as opposed to being in discrete patches. Inflammation occurs at the basis of the Crypts of Lieberkühn, damaging new epithelial cells and causing abscesses to form.

Epithelial ulceration and sloughing of the mucosa result. As mucosal repair is attempted, highly vascularised granulation tissue covers the lumen of the bowel, giving a velvety red appearance of superficial ulcers (on endoscopy) and a friable texture. These changes only affect the mucosa and submucosa, except in rare, acute cases when the muscularis is eroded and perforation occurs.

Proposed causes

The cause is unkown, although the following have been implicated:

- an immunological response to antigens
- diet (reduced fibre or milk).

Stress is not thought to be a cause but may exacerbate the symptoms (Rhodes & Mayberry 1986).

Symptoms

Bloody diarrhoea characterises ulcerative colitis. This is associated with frequency, urgency and abdominal cramps which are relieved by defaecation. There may also be pus in the stools and blood loss may vary from being mild to causing shock. In severe attacks, patients will feel exhausted and may suffer weight loss and anorexia.

Related manifestations

People with ulcerative colitis may also experience associated extracolonic problems, including:

- *Arthritis* (large joints) – this is becoming less common now sulphasalazine is used for maintenance therapy
- *Ankylosing spondylitis* – abnormal consolidation and immobility of the bones in the vertebral joints; ankylosing spondylitis and ulcerative colitis appear to be linked genetically
- *Erythema nodosum* – red painful lumps on the lower legs, shins and occasionally the arms, which may develop during a relapse but which tend to settle once in remission
- *Pyoderma gangrenosum* – chronic skin ulceration occurring on the extremities
- *Iritis* – inflammation of the iris causing pain, photophobia, contraction of the pupil and discolouration of the iris
- *Episcleritis* – inflammation of the eyeball
- *Primary sclerosing cholangitis* – fibrosing process of the biliary tract leading to cirrhosis. This affects 2–3% of sufferers; 80% of primary sclerosing cholangitis sufferers have ulcerative colitis (Travis et al 1993).

Extra-intestinal manifestations, except for ankylosing spondylitis, hepatobiliary disease and in some cases pyoderma gangrenosum, are relieved when the bowel is removed surgically.

Other complications to be considered are perforation of the bowel during a severe attack and the increased incidence of colonic cancer in people with long-standing ulcerative colitis, although it may be less common than originally thought (see Ch. 7). Regular colonoscopies (i.e. every second year) may be offered to sufferers who have pancolitis and who had symptoms for over 10 years, the frequency being adjusted if abnormalities are noted.

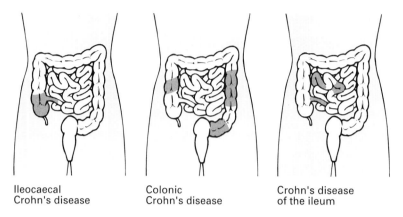

| Ileocaecal Crohn's disease | Colonic Crohn's disease | Crohn's disease of the ileum |

Fig 3.3   Areas affected in Crohn's disease.

Crohn's disease

Crohn's disease is an inflammatory disorder which affects any part of the gastrointestinal tract from the lips to the anus, but most commonly the distal ileum and proximal colon (see Fig. 3.3). One of the distinguishing features compared to ulcerative colitis is that the areas affected are skip lesions, i.e. they are interrupted by areas of healthy tissue. This phenomenon remains unexplained, as does the cause of the illness.

Crohn's disease is also characterised by remission and relapse, with periods of remission lasting up to five years. There is no cure, but prompt intervention can decrease damage and complications, induce remission, repair strictures or remove severely damaged or perforated sections of gut.

Incidence and prevalence

- Usually first diagnosed in young adults but can also occur in childhood and later years
- Affects both sexes about equally
- Affects western Caucasians of European Anglo-Saxon descent, but is uncommon elsewhere in the world. Jews of European descent have a higher incidence than corresponding non-Jewish Caucasians
- 30–500/100 000 of the population are affected and five new cases/100 000 are diagnosed each year
- 15% have a relative with an inflammatory bowel disease
- It is four times more common in smokers than in non-smokers, in contrast to ulcerative colitis
- Since 1950 the incidence of Crohn's disease has doubled (Travis et al 1993).

Pathology

Disease may arise anywhere in the alimentary tract, 90% of patients having involvement of the terminal ileum. Inflammation extends through the entire thickness of the bowel wall, with oedema, granulomata and giant cells. Lymph nodes are involved and the extent of inflammation causes fissures which may become fistulae or abscesses. As ulceration progresses, the bowel becomes thickened and stenosed with strictures narrowing the lumen of the gut. As the serosa become inflamed, there is a tendency for affected loops of bowel to 'stick' to other structures, including affected or unaffected bowel, adjacent organs or the abdominal wall. On examination, there are deep fissured ulcers and a 'cobblestone' appearance to the mucosa.

Proposed causes

Once again, the cause is unknown but the following have been implicated:

- genetic susceptibility to an unknown antigen
- infective agents
- a diet that is high in refined sugars.

Symptoms

Initially, these may be vague and occasional, and so the patient may not have a diagnosis for years. Symptoms depend on the site of ulceration but commonly include malaise, anorexia and abdominal pain, which can settle in the right iliac fossa and is often severe. In patients with partial obstruction, pain is crampy and intermittent but an acute exacerbation will be associated with severe, persistent pain and abdominal tenderness, possibly with fistula or abscess formation. Diarrhoea is a consistent sign and, unlike ulcerative colitis, it is unlikely to be bloody. In partial obstruction, the patient may experience vomiting and intermittent diarrhoea or no bowel movement at all.

The other common tell-tale sign is the presence of anal or perianal lesions, either alone as a forerunner of the diagnosis or in association with abdominal symptoms.

Related manifestations

In common with ulcerative colitis, about 15% of sufferers develop problems with other organs and joints. These include:

- arthritis – with large bowel disease
- ankylosing spondylitis – affects 6% of sufferers
- sacroiliitis – inflammation of the sacrum and the ilium (haunch bone); affects 16% of sufferers
- erythema nodosum
- pyoderma gangrenosum
- apthous ulcers – thrush-like ulcers in the mouth
- iritis and episcleritis
- finger clubbing
- gallstones – affect people with ileal disease or ileal resections due to malabsorption of bile salts; this is very common
- psychiatric disorders.

Other complications that should be considered are small bowel obstruction, toxic dilation of the large bowel and perforation. Abscesses may occur either in the abdomen, pelvis or the ischiorectal connective tissue. There may also be an increased risk of developing cancer (Travis et al 1993).

DIAGNOSIS

Generally the symptoms of inflammatory bowel disease are embarrassing, worrying and socially unacceptable to the sufferer. As a result, many patients modify their lifestyle to accommodate such symptoms for some considerable time prior to seeking medical assistance. Once medical assistance is sought, it is important to investigate the patient's symptoms promptly, to alleviate their fears. It is hoped this will establish a diagnosis, and the extent and severity of the disease, noting any complications associated with the disease, and ultimately allowing treatment to begin. The distinction between ulcerative colitis and Crohn's disease is vital for patients with colitis, as treatment options will differ according to diagnosis.

The investigations conducted will be determined by the patient's specific symptoms and a detailed history, but diagnosis is achieved by considering history and the results on endoscopy, contrast radiology and histopathology together. Most patients are seen, have investigations and are given diagnosis and treatment options as outpatients – it is the minority who are immediately admitted as in-patients, or who are diagnosed after having been admitted.

The investigations conducted for patients with suspected ulcerative colitis or Crohn's disease are invasive and uncomfortable for the patient and they can also be embarrassing. They are also physically and psychologically demanding for the patient who is already feeling unwell.

Many patients have little idea about what is expected of them when they arrive in the hospital for investigation. To alleviate any fears, it is important to ensure that any queries and anxieties are addressed by providing information in private. This can be assisted by assessing the patient's psychological state of mind. Ideally, education should be commenced via the general practitioner, gastroenterologist, nurse specialist or ward staff.

Diagnosis brings with it mixed responses. In general, patients are relieved to have an identified cause for their symptoms. Many feel justified in feeling so ill and are eager to be treated promptly. Relief at having a diagnosis other than cancer is often expressed. Alternatively, patients often express concern at what a diagnosis of ulcerative colitis or Crohn's disease involves. Many patients will have relatives, friends or colleagues who have inflammatory bowel disease, or will know of a sufferer. As a result, second-hand information is passed along to the patient. Unfortunately, this information can be inaccurate and out of date, leaving the patient confused and misinformed.

History

When taking the history, the following should be noted:

1. stool frequency, especially presence of blood
2. frequency and severity of abdominal pain
3. any changes in weight
4. assessment of the patient's appetite and dietary intake, noting condition of the mouth
5. signs of fatigue and malaise

6. duration of symptoms
7. extra-intestinal signs.

Bowel habit

A more detailed history of bowel habit, including frequency and whether stools are bloody or not, is important. Frequency of bloody stools is a principal sign of the severity of colitis in ulcerative colitis patients. During a relapse, a stool specimen may be tested for

- microbiology, culture and sensitivity
- *Clostridium difficile* toxin assay, to exclude an infective cause for symptoms.

The appearance of the stool should be noted, observing for pus, blood, mucus and the consistency. In-patients should have the volume, appearance and frequency of stool monitored to indicate the severity of disease and its response to treatment.

Physical examination

Physical examination of the abdomen will be conducted to note any guarding, tenderness, masses, old scars or fistulae. An examination of the anal/rectal area for any skin tags, fistulae, and general skin condition will be carried out.

Endoscopy

A sigmoidoscopy involves examining the rectum and sigmoid colon with a rigid or fibre-optic instrument called a sigmoidoscope. The general condition of the mucosa is noted and biopsies may be taken. A flexible sigmoidoscopy achieves examination potential to the splenic flexure, while a rigid sigmoidoscopy only extends to the sigmoid colon.

Physical preparation of the patient

A phosphate enema may be given before the procedure to clear the rectum and lower end of the sigmoid colon of faeces. This allows a clearer view of the mucosa. However, this procedure may be conducted as an emergency without any preparation if the rectum is empty. If biopsies are taken, nurses will check for sudden rectal bleeding after the procedure, and warn the patient that some bleeding may occur.

Colonoscopy

Colonoscopy is performed to examine the entire colon and rectum, almost always under sedation. The appearance of the colonic mucosa is examined and biopsies are taken if required.

Preparation

Preparation of the bowel to enable a successful colonoscopy is vital. The presence of even small particles of faecal matter may obscure abnormal mucosa from the endoscopist's view. To avoid the patient having to have another colonoscopy (and prepare for it), thorough bowel preparation is vital. This is achieved by restricting diet to a low residue or clear fluid intake only on the day before the colonoscopy. Various purgatives may be prescribed for the patient to take the day before the procedure, the choice being dependent on the following factors:

- consultant's preference
- underlying disease
- patient's age and general health
- time available for preparation
- availability.

Whatever product is chosen, it is vital that the patient is clearly advised about developing diarrhoea and to drink significant fluids in order not to become dehydrated and for preparation to be effective. The patient will also benefit from being informed that the preparation is the worst aspect of the procedure, but vital for its success.

Other aspects of preparation include:

- Baseline observations, pulse and blood pressure are recorded so that abnormalities can be noted after the procedure.
- Informed consent to the procedure must be gained from the patient; hence a thorough explanation must be given of what is to happen and what will be required.
- The patient should be starved for 4 h before the procedure to prevent the risk of aspiration whilst sedated.
- An intravenous cannula must be placed in position for the administration of sedation.
- The patient is asked to wear a gown to prevent soiling of their clothes.
- Moreover, the patient will be advised to stop taking iron supplements or antacid preparations 7 days prior to the procedure, as these preparations are difficult to clear out of the bowel. If the bowel contains these preparations the endoscopist will have difficulty examining the condition of the mucosa.

Recovery

The patient is drowsy following the procedure and should be allowed to sleep off the sedation before being offered a drink. Observations of pulse, blood pressure and respiratory rate must be recorded regularly ($\frac{1}{2}$–1 hourly) until the patient is awake and observations are stable. This is to detect any abnormalities, noting the risk of perforation to the bowel or oversedation.

Patients who are having a colonoscopy as an outpatient should have a relative or friend to drive them home.

Radiology

Barium enema

This shows the outline of the ileum, colon and rectum. Abnormalities, including an irregular ulcerated mucosa, polyps, tumours or diverticula, may be seen with a double-contrast barium enema. Barium is introduced per rectum, the patient is encouraged to move around whilst lying down, and then gas is introduced into the bowel for the double contrast. In addition to bowel preparation, patients need to be warned that this is a very undignified experience.

Preparation. As for colonoscopy, the colon must be empty for accurate pictures/results and a bowel purgative regime will be prescribed. The patient may drink clear fluid up to the time of the procedure as they will not be sedated.

Recovery. The only specific advice is to inform patients that their stools will be pale initially after the test, due to the barium. They should be advised to continue to drink plenty of fluid to maintain transit of stool and barium through the colon and rectum.

Barium swallow and follow-through
This shows the small bowel on X-ray with barium contrast, outlining 'cobblestone' mucosa or strictures characteristic of Crohn's disease. The patient drinks the barium and a series of pictures are taken over 4–6 h as it progresses through the ileum.

Small bowel enema
This achieves the same result as the barium swallow and follow-through, but in a shorter time (up to 1 h). Barium is introduced via a nasoduodenal tube and a series of pictures are taken as described above.

Preparation of the patient. The day before the procedure the patient requires a low residue diet. At 1600 h, the patient is required to take 40 ml of magnesium sulphate with a warm drink, followed by clear fluids only.

Recovery of the patient. Patients may eat and drink immediately after the procedure. It should be noted that the preparation and recovery of the patient may vary slightly depending upon where and by whom the investigation is conducted.

Blood tests
1. Erythrocyte sedimentation rate (ESR) and C-reactive protein (CRP) are measured, as these will usually be raised during acute inflammation.
2. Full blood count is taken to look for anaemia, as the patient may experience overt or occult gastrointestinal bleeding. A raised white cell count may indicate infection.
3. Urea and electrolyte (U & E) levels enable the assessment of fluid and electrolyte imbalance.

Psychological effect of initial diagnosis
Common anxieties and concerns expressed by patients when a diagnosis is made include: 'Will I take steroids for ever?'; 'Having to wear a bag for the rest of my life!'; 'How real is the threat of cancer?'

Drossman et al (1991) have addressed the issue of patients' concerns and anxieties in relation to IBD. In providing a list of patient worries, it is interesting to note that patients with ulcerative colitis and Crohn's disease rank their anxieties differently, just as the pathophysiological characteristics of the two

Table 3.1 Disease-related concerns in Crohn's disease and ulcerative colitis

Crohn's disease	Ulcerative colitis
Uncertain nature of disease	Having a stoma bag
Energy level	Developing cancer
Effect of medication	Effect of medication
Having surgery	Uncertain nature of disease
Having a stoma bag	Having surgery
Being a burden on others	Energy level

conditions are different (see Table 3.1). Collectively, the first five patient concerns are:

1. uncertain nature of disease
2. effect of medication
3. energy level
4. having surgery
5. having a stoma bag.

Drossman et al (1991) also noted that patient concerns can affect the course and outcome of their treatment. Patients' concerns and lack of knowledge will influence:

1. contentment with their care
2. adjustment to their illness
3. structure of treatment
4. compliance to treatment.

Although Drossman et al (1991) based their work within the American health care system, it is suggested that the concerns and worries highlighted are a valid starting point on which to focus patient education in the UK. Specific fears personal to each patient come to light through assessing the patient's existing knowledge and understanding of the situation they find themselves in, and through counselling of patients. As a result, specific relevant information can be provided. Verbal information is ideally supported by literature, videos or audio tapes to guide and inform clients and their families in the comfort and privacy of their own home. Care should be taken to ensure that supplementary information supports what clinicians have said, and will say, to patients. Because misinformation can be worse than no information, it is important to ensure that patients are guided towards material that is appropriate for them.

Compliance and understanding of treatment may also be improved by employing the principles of 'self-medication'. By informing patients about the purpose, storage, dosage, side-effects, administration, precautions and specific information regarding their medication, they will improve their technique and accuracy of administering their drugs which may ultimately result in improved health (Bird & Hassal 1993). To enhance and develop the information provided to patients, it is important not to neglect the work of other disciplines, e.g. stoma therapy nurse, dietician, social worker, pharmacist and support agencies such as the National Association for Colitis and Crohn's disease (NACC) and Crohn's in Childhood Research Association (CICRA).

MISDIAGNOSIS

Misdiagnosis, unfortunately, is not uncommon and can have devastating effects, particularly if Crohn's disease is misdiagnosed as ulcerative colitis. It is not only problematic because the symptoms experienced by the patient are unrelieved and treated inappropriately, but it also leaves the patient feeling frustrated and confused when symptoms do not improve. Often patients feel undervalued and discredited when their symptoms persist. Conditions diagnosed in the place of inflammatory bowel disease are both physical and psychological in nature (see Case history 3.1). These include:

- irritable bowel syndrome
- bleeding haemorrhoids
- anxiety states
- gastroenteritis
- gynaecological causes
- anorexia nervosa (Kelly 1992).

Case history 3.1

Martha first contacted her general practitioner when she was 12 years old, complaining of mouth ulcers, weight loss, vomiting and diarrhoea. Investigations carried out over a period of a year, including blood tests, an endoscopy, barium meal and a bone marrow aspirate, failed to find a physical cause to explain the symptoms. As a result, Martha was interviewed by a psychiatrist and a diagnosis of anorexia nervosa was made. Martha was admitted to an adolescent centre where she was locked in a single room. All her property was removed, and phone calls and letters were not permitted. Communication from friends and relatives was considered a luxury that was allowed only in response to weight gain. Throughout her admission to the unit, Martha continued to experience weight loss, diarrhoea and nausea. The staff's beliefs that Martha was suffering from anorexia nervosa were reinforced because she often vomited after eating. Bed rest was enforced as a way to reserve energy, and a bed pan was provided as a toilet. After a period of 3 months, Martha was able to escape to her sister's in Glasgow. Trying to rebuild her life, Martha applied and was accepted to train as a nursery nurse. Having commenced her training, Martha's new general practitioner referred her to a local gastroenterologist. After further investigations, including a small bowel examination, an endoscopy, a colonoscopy and further blood tests, a diagnosis of Crohn's disease was made. When Martha was finally diagnosed, she was 16 years of age and weighed 22 kg (three and a half stones).

Once the cycle of misdiagnosis and inappropriate treatment commences, the client begins to lose faith and trust in the practitioners with whom they come into contact. As a result, patients who have been misdiagnosed require a great deal of support and reassurance once the correct diagnosis is established and appropriate treatment commenced.

OUTPATIENT CARE

Because of the nature of inflammatory bowel disease, the majority of sufferers can be managed solely as outpatients, never requiring hospitalisation. Visiting an outpatient clinic can be a very daunting experience. The sufferer has to deal with the news that they have a chronic, often incurable disorder which is potentially highly embarrassing and degrading. This is made worse by having to discuss the symptoms and problems with other people, often total strangers.

During a visit to the clinic, the patient will be weighed to ascertain gains or losses and may have access to a dietician for assessment and advice. An up-to-date summary of the signs and symptoms will be obtained and a rigid sigmoidoscopy will usually be performed if the patient has symptoms of an exacerbation. Biopsies may also be taken. Throughout the consultation, the patient's privacy must be observed and considered.

If the sufferer sees a familiar face at the clinic, this may help to relieve some of the anxieties. An inflammatory bowel disease or gastroenterology nurse specialist may provide the answer to this, as in a large hospital it is not always practical or possible for a patient to see the same doctor on each visit to the clinic.

The nurse specialist can provide the clinic attenders with the pastoral care made possible by consistent contact and with practical information, i.e. leaflets, books, videos. The role has the scope for expansion, with the clinical nurse specialist possibly being responsible for clinics alongside medical practitioners both in the base hospital and in surrounding areas (satellite clinics). Ideally, the patients would have direct access to their nurse specialist and be able to drop in to a clinic or contact them by telephone whenever they feel the need. In reality, this may prove difficult.

Recommendations for the role of the inflammatory bowel disease nurse specialist include:

- nurse-led clinics in the base hospital and surrounding areas, the nurse thus becoming a link between the community and the hospital
- counselling service for newly diagnosed patients and their families
- link between other disciplines, e.g. stoma nurses, social workers, dieticians and support groups
- educational resource for patients and staff
- conducting relaxation classes for sufferers.

Drug treatment

Because the cause of inflammatory bowel disease is unknown, drugs are used therapeutically to achieve remission and then maintain it, thus improving the sufferer's quality of life. Patients will need to know that symptoms usually respond to drug therapy.

Corticosteroids – prednisolone and hydrocortisone

These constitute the first line of treatment for acute attacks and relapses from remission. In acutely ill patients, hydrocortisone is administered intravenously and rectally for ulcerative colitis. Alternatively, prednisolone can be prescribed orally and/or rectally in the form of foam or liquid enemas, which patients require help and instruction to administer. Side-effects and the importance of following reducing dose regimens need to be understood by patients upon commencing a course of oral steroids. Usually, steroids are given for some weeks, reduced over a defined period and then stopped, providing symptoms do not return.

5-Amino salicylic acid – compounds

These are used to maintain remission and to reduce the frequency of relapse. Sulphasalazine is used in ulcerative colitis and colonic Crohn's disease. Mesalazine is available as Asacol capsules which rupture in the small bowel and are effective when treating ulcerative colitis. Pentasa comes in the form of granules in a special coating that dissolves in the duodenum so the drug is slowly liberated as it passes down the gut. This is used when treating Crohn's disease in the upper gut.

Immunosuppressants – azathioprine

These are used for steroid-dependent disease, i.e. in those patients whose symptoms return as the steroid dose is reduced. Evidence of their effectiveness in achieving remission is stronger in Crohn's disease than in ulcerative colitis.

Support agencies

NACC (National Association for Colitis and Crohn's disease) is a registered charity and is extremely active in promoting support for sufferers and conducting research into IBD. NACC provides free booklets regarding IBD to members, both patients and medical personnel alike. Practical help for sufferers includes local support groups and a 'can't wait' card (Fig. 3.4) to help patients gain access to toilets (see Useful Addresses on p. 84).

IN-PATIENT CARE

The value of nursing

Patients who are admitted to hospital can expect to have a named nurse to take responsibility for and coordinate their care (Department of Health 1995). This goal can be achieved through using a variety of methods of allocating nursing staff. One way of promoting valuable nursing care is to adopt the philosophy of primary nursing, organised within a team of nurses. The benefits of using primary nursing with patients suffering from IBD include the following:

- One nurse coordinates the patient's care throughout their hospital admission.

NATIONAL ASSOCIATION for COLITIS and CROHN'S DISEASE

A registered National Charity No. 282732

PLEASE HELP

Due to an illness, which is not infectious, our member needs toilet facilities urgently.

THANK YOU

Fig 3.4   A 'can't wait' card, supplied by the NACC.

- The risk of cross-infection is reduced, as fewer nurses care for the patient.
- With a small group of nurses caring for a patient, there are fewer people for the patient to become embarrassed in front of when intimate care is required, e.g. administering enemas.
- Through caring for a patient on a regular basis, the named nurse can develop a trusting, honest and understanding relationship with the client. Consequently, the primary nurse can anticipate patient needs and provide effective empathy and support whilst empowering clients to become active in their own care through education, commitment and instilling confidence. With repeated admissions, the patient's nurse can extend the relationship by updating patient assessments rather than covering old ground, thus advancing the continuity of patient care.
- A family-centred approach to care is developed as the family of the patient becomes familiar with the primary nurse and involved in the patient's care.

Unfortunately, when the medical management of IBD fails and surgical intervention is required, this usually means a move for the patient to the surgical unit. Ideally, the medical and surgical units could be combined to promote continuity of care by the primary nurse, thus reducing the patient's anxiety about moving wards, increasing nursing skills and knowledge in caring for patients with both medical and surgical problems and increasing job satisfaction for nurses.

Severe attack of inflammatory bowel disease requiring hospitalisation

A severe attack which does not respond to oral steroids will necessitate the sufferer being admitted to hospital for an intensive regime of intravenous therapy. The gut is rested by starving the patient and the inflammation is reduced by administering intravenous steroids (and, for patients with ulcerative colitis, rectal steroids as well) for about 5 days. Dehydration and any electrolyte imbalance is corrected with intravenous fluids (approximately

3 L / day). Crohn's disease sufferers will usually be prescribed metronidazole as they may have an associated infection which is difficult to differentiate from inflammation.

The progress and response to treatment are monitored by:

- stool frequency and consistency
- temperature and pulse rate
- patterns of FBC, ESR and CRP
- the patient's attitude towards how they are feeling
- pain
- anorexia
- response to reintroducing diet.

The nurse's role
This can be defined as follows:

- ensuring the patient is kept well-informed and up-to-date with their progress and treatment according to their understanding, whilst aiming to relieve anxiety.
- encouraging the patient to become involved in their own care, i.e. administering their own rectal steroids, completing their own fluid and stool charts.
- recording the patient's vital signs four times a day, reporting any pronounced changes to the medical staff as they may indicate early signs of perforation. It should be remembered that these signs may be masked by the steroids. The value of accurate stool charts cannot be underestimated as stool frequency and type are the main criteria for deciding further treatment options.
- ensuring the patient is referred to the stoma therapist at an early stage as surgery may be implicated if the flare-up does not respond to this course of treatment. Although this may seem a radical move, in the long term, patients benefit greatly by having the time to digest this information, and it thus enables them to accept surgery if necessary.
- considering the patient's hygiene needs, encouraging daily baths and providing a barrier cream to prevent excoriation of the skin during episodes of frequent diarrhoea. Oral hygiene also needs consideration while the patient is fasting.
- encouraging rest periods throughout the day if the patient is very lethargic or tired. This may be due to anaemia as a result of the blood loss incurred during an exacerbation. Nurses may find they need to negotiate appropriate numbers of visitors and time and duration of their stay according to how the patient is feeling and the need to rest.
- ensuring the patient receives adequate analgesia, by encouraging the patient to vocalise about their pain, describing its site, nature and severity. It should be remembered that some of these patients endure chronic pain, so they may not exhibit the expected body language when they are in discomfort and their pain should not therefore be written off as imaginary or be ignored.

A pain thermometer or other assessment tool can be used both before and after administration of analgesia, e.g. a pain score scale:

- score 1 – no pain on movement or rest
- score 2 – slight pain on movement, little pain at rest
- score 3 – moderate pain on movement, slight pain at rest
- score 4 – severe pain on movement, moderate pain at rest
- score 5 – excruciating pain on movement or rest.

The analgesia used may be an antispasmodic agent or opiate-based. A patient-controlled analgesia pump (PCA) may be considered during the acute stage of an exacerbation. The PCA allows the patient to promote their own comfort and more importantly permits additional boluses of analgesia if the spasmodic pain returns, i.e. on defaecation. In addition, the PCA can address constant pain by using a background infusion. Some patients, however, do not wish to control their own analgesia or do not have the dexterity to do so. When using a PCA pump, it is suggested that a monitoring chart is used to ensure the safety of the patient. In patients with ulcerative colitis, opiates should be avoided because they may promote toxic dilatation. Fortunately, they are rarely necessary, unlike in Crohn's disease when obstructive pain is severe and is only relieved by opiates.

Some patients gain a great deal of relief from localised pain by using a heat pad. Most patients will respond completely or partially to intensive medical treatment (Travis et al 1993).

If remission does not appear imminent with an intravenous regime, the medical staff may decide to introduce intravenous cyclosporin. However, if, despite intensive medical intervention, the patient fails to improve or if their condition deteriorates, surgery will be indicated.

Surgical intervention
The operation performed depends upon:

- diagnosis
- site of disease
- urgency of surgical intervention
- patient's general condition
- existing/potential complications
- previous surgery
- patient's wishes.

Surgery is generally used as a last resort when medical management fails, since it carries with it potential complications:

- infection
- adhesions
- paralytic ileus
- breakdown of anastamosis
- diarrhoea
- malabsorption and dietary problems
- complications associated with stoma formation (see Chapter 9).

Whilst approaches to medical management of both Crohn's disease and ulcerative colitis patients are similar, surgical interventions differ according to the patient's diagnosis, and thus are considered separately. Either group may develop complications associated with abdominal surgery postoperatively.

Surgery for patients with Crohn's disease

Emergency laparotomy and resection of diseased bowel. This may involve the small bowel or the colon and/or the rectum. If the affected bowel is dilated and toxic, a stoma is more likely to be made than a direct end-to-end anastamosis.

Proctocolectomy and ileostomy formation. Resection of the entire colon and rectum with formation of an ileostomy. The anus and a rectal stump may be left in situ if not diseased.

Colectomy and ileorectal anastamosis. Resection of the colon and end-to-end anastamosis of the ileum to the rectum. Patients pass liquid stools with increased frequency postoperatively. Over months or years, the consistency may thicken a little and the frequency may decrease. Patients with Crohn's colitis which require resection usually have the entire colon and rectum removed because there is usually more than one ulcerative lesion in the colon. Pouch surgery is not appropriate as Crohn's lesions are likely to arise in the pouch and cause severe problems (see p. 74).

Formation of ileostomy. In this case, the affected part of the bowel distal from the stoma is 'rested' by diverting the faecal stream through an ileostomy. The stoma may be either an end ileostomy with separate mucous fistula or a loop ileostomy. This is a relatively common surgical intervention for patients with Crohn's colitis and facilitates topical application of steroid enemas to the distal section of bowel. These are administered via a catheter inserted either into the distal loop of a loop ileostomy or into the mucous fistula. If and when remission is achieved, the ileostomy may be closed.

Strictureplasty. This is particularly used in patients with previous small bowel disease. Narrowed/strictured areas of the ileum are 'refashioned' to restore the lumen of the gut and relieve obstruction without resecting large lengths of small bowel.

Surgery for patients with ulcerative colitis

Unlike those with Crohn's disease, patients with ulcerative colitis who require surgery always have proctectomy (removal of the rectum) as this is where disease arises and where it will recur if a stump or remnant is left in situ. This alters the surgical options available for this group of patients.

Emergency laparotomy and resection of colon and rectum. This necessitates stoma formation. The anal sphincter is likely to be left in situ with options for future surgery to be considered after emergency period.

Proctectomy. Removal of the rectum and formation of colostomy, if it has not already been done.

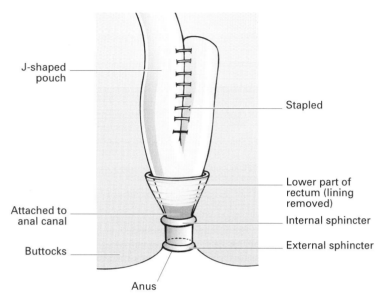

J-shaped pouch

Stapled

Lower part of rectum (lining removed)

Attached to anal canal

Internal sphincter

Buttocks

External sphincter

Anus

Fig 3.5   Proctocolectomy and formation of an ileo-anal pouch.

Panproctocolectomy. Excision of the entire colon and rectum and ileostomy formation.

Proctocolectomy and formation of ileo-anal pouch. The colon and rectum are removed, and then a reservoir or 'pouch' is formed using the ileum. This is joined to the anus above the sphincter (see Fig. 3.5). Usually an ileostomy is formed to facilitate healing of the pouch, and the stoma is reversed at a later date. Patients now effectively have a reservoir in which liquid stool collects, which can be emptied by relaxing the anal sphincter in the usual way. Over months and years, stool consistency thickens and the frequency of emptying reduces as the ileal pouch and pelvic muscles adapt.

Considerations relating to ileo-anal pouch surgery. At first glance this option may seem to be preferable for all patients with ulcerative colitis who require proctocolectomy. However, it involves lengthy, complex surgery which will have major effects on the patient's future life, and an understanding of what is involved is vital before any decisions are made.

Whilst a few, very fit patients may be able to undergo the entire procedure in one operation, these people are exceptional and most patients have two or three separate operations over several months. This involves having an ileostomy, albeit temporarily, repeated hospital admissions and visits, and repeated exposure to the risks associated with surgery.

For pouch surgery to be appropriate, the patient needs to have good anal sphincter control, as incontinence will result otherwise. A good nutritional state and being physically fit prior to commencing surgery are vital to withstand the rigours of recovery and re-training bowel habit.

Pre-operatively, patients require specific information and counselling about pouch surgery, as well as general advice given to patients having planned abdominal surgery. Specific areas include:

- the anatomy and refashioning involved
- implications of pouch formation on bowel habit
- the need to empty the pouch as often as 2-hourly, day and night, in the initial stages of its use and adapting to it
- the potential for faeces and / or flatus leaking from the pouch
- the need for anorectal physiology studies to test sphincter pressures and strength
- ileostomy siting, formation and subsequent care with meeting stoma nurse therapist
- meeting a patient who has experienced pouch surgery to provide information and an opportunity to share and discuss fears or concerns.

Postoperative care is as for any patient having surgery on the small bowel. In addition, the following specific points are important:

- *Care of rectal drain* – this drain is designed to clear the pouch of old blood and is kept patent by flushing it slowly twice daily with 30 ml of saline from the first postoperative day. It is removed after 4 or 5 days, once bile-stained stool is passed through the drain. Once the rectal drain is removed, patients are advised to use a barrier cream after opening their pouch, in order to protect the surrounding skin and prevent excoriation.

- The patient is advised to 'empty' their pouch 2-hourly (including at night) initially. Patients liken this to severe flare-up of their ulcerative colitis. Time and perseverance will result in them recognising when they need to empty their pouch, and the frequency will reduce. Some clients experience leakage from their newly formed pouch when relaxed in bed at night or during sexual intercourse. Clients should be advised to empty their pouch before going to bed or prior to intercourse and initially to wear a pad during the night. This will improve as the ileal mucosa in the pouch adapts and pelvic muscles adapt to pouch function over the course of the first year.

- *Diet* – once the rectal drain has been removed the patient can begin to take fluids orally. This is built up slowly over the next 24–48 hours when a soft diet is commenced. Again this is added to slowly until a normal diet can be resumed.

Dietary tastes and preferences are extremely individual. However, there are some specific hints regarding the patient's bowel function which can be helpful.

- Begin by eating small meals; this will prevent a bloated feeling.
- Try adding different foods to the diet singly. This will help the patient to identify which foods affect their bowel function, for example:
  — cheese, potatoes, pasta and bananas may decrease pouch output
  — beans, alcohol, caffeine, spicy foods and wholemeal foods may increase pouch output

— onions, sweetcorn, green vegetables, beans and milk may increase flatus

— spicy foods, grapefruit, nuts, popcorn and salad may increase anal irritation

— potato skins, tomatoes and nuts have been associated with blocking the flow into the pouch (Meadows et al 1994, Jameson 1992)

• Referral to support agencies is important to provide encouragement, education and advice for patients. These groups are generally connected to the specialist centres performing the surgery (for example The Kangaroo Club, The Plymouth Possums).

Complications associated with pouch surgery specifically may occur in the immediate postoperative phases, after pouch formation or ileostomy reversal, or months or years later. Patients need to be aware of this possibility to be able to respond appropriately (see Table 3.2). Overall, complication rates vary. They seem generally to be associated with the expertise of the team involved and with whether or not the patient has a 'covering' ileostomy.

Nurse's role

Whether an emergency colectomy is performed or surgery is planned, it is the nurse's role to coordinate care and prepare the client physically and psychologically for their operation. If an emergency colectomy is indicated, preoperative care can be limited, but additional information can be given between surgical procedures. Wherever possible, it is helpful to introduce the

Table 3.2 Complications associated with pouch surgery

Problem	Likely time of occurrence
Wound sepsis	More likely in the weeks and months after surgery
Pelvic sepsis: haematoma or leakage from anastamosis	More likely in the weeks and months after surgery
Pouch/pelvic abscess	More likely in the weeks and months after surgery
Fistula formation	More likely in the weeks and months after surgery
Anastamosis breakdown	More likely in the weeks and months after surgery
Pouchitis	Can occur up to 5 years after surgery
Dehydration due to fluid and electrolyte loss	At any time
Incontinence of flatus and/or faeces	Onset within weeks/months – worse at night
Sore anus and perianal sites	Can occur at any time
Strictures at anastamoses sites	Develops over months postoperatively
Intestinal obstruction	More common in patients with temporary ileostomy
Urinary problems	More common in women than men
Sexual dysfunction	More likely in the months after surgery

patient to surgical staff pre-operatively. They will have the opportunity to discuss procedures and expectations with surgeons and nurses directly responsible for their care.

Pre-operative care

Pre-operative care for patients with Crohn's disease or ulcerative colitis is the same as for any patient having abdominal surgery.

To be able to provide informed consent the patient requires:

- information about anatomy and physiology and proposed changes
- expected outcomes
- possible complications
- siting of a stoma by a stoma therapist or suitably experienced nurse and opportunities to discuss the future as regards life with stoma
- introduction to another patient who has undergone similar surgery; this is often helpful for education and alleviation of any fears or worries the patient may be experiencing.

A patient also requires physiotherapy referral for teaching of deep breathing and leg exercises.

Some patients travel from other parts of the country to specialist centres for their surgery. Nursing staff can make their stay more comfortable by considering adopting relaxed visiting hours, arranging accommodation at the hospital, or providing a list of reasonably priced accommodation in the area for friends and relatives. Additionally, as patients may well be off work for some considerable time before and after surgery is performed, a social worker may be able to provide useful advice on benefits and travelling expenses.

Time must be spent discussing the patient's fears and anxieties. Patients are grateful for any relevant information provided and need to be informed to be able to become involved in their care and recovery. Nurses are in a good position to provide this support as they can generally make the time and resources to coordinate care and counsel patients.

Postoperative care

The patient will receive routine care similar to that given following a laparotomy. The patient can expect to have an intravenous infusion, urinary catheter, drains into the abdomen and possibly an epidural infusion, PCA and a nasogastric tube in position on return from theatre. Once nasogastric drainage is minimal and bowel sounds have resumed, fluids can be taken orally. Intake is gradually increased as tolerated until the patient can manage a normal diet.

Routine stoma care is given as required (see Ch. 4) and prophylactic antibiotics are given immediately postoperatively.

As with other abdominal surgery, patients are advised not to lift heavy objects for 3–6 months, or to drive until they can safely perform an emergency stop. When driving one needs to be able to make sudden, forceful leg movements in confidence without automatic inhibition from pain or strain on abdominal wounds and muscles.

Returning to work depends upon the patient's type of work and their general health. Patients will experience fatigue on their discharge. They should be advised to rest, take gentle exercise and eat a well-balanced diet.

Privacy

Patients entering hospital for medical management of their inflammatory bowel disease can find the whole experience humiliating and depressing. Experiencing incontinence and the use of commodes behind curtains within a mixed ward are unacceptable. Patients should be cared for, wherever possible, within a single sex ward or bay or ideally in a single room with en suite toilet facilities. Curtains dividing patients offer no privacy from smell, sound or unwanted visitors (Buswell 1993). Single rooms with en suite toilet facilities offer privacy for personal hygiene, the administering of enemas, the sound and smell of frequent defaecation, education and discussions regarding diagnosis and treatment, and finally provide an environment in which families can give support and emotional care through touch and intimacy. The use of single rooms allows clients to embark on their treatment with the minimum fear of embarrassment.

To ensure privacy is respected, 'do not disturb' signs can be displayed outside the room. The provision of single sex toilet and washing facilities goes some way to avoiding embarrassment and upholding the patient's dignity.

Boredom

Patients admitted to hospital for management of their ulcerative colitis or Crohn's disease find themselves resident for periods of days, and occasionally weeks or months. After a short time, patients find the experience tedious and monotonous. The days are long and mainly uneventful, particularly if the day is not interrupted by meals. To try to relieve these feelings of boredom and frustration, nurses can encourage the use of the hospital facilities, possibly with the help and support of family and friends to facilitate access.

These include:

- television/video
- radio/hospital radio
- literature
- hospital chaplain
- volunteer manicurist/hairdresser
- the hospital grounds.

Not only do these distractions help entertain patients, but they can also provide additional activities so that attention is moved away from their illness and pain. An open visiting policy is beneficial, as patients can have family and friends visiting throughout the day. However, nurses must be aware of the needs of tired patients who are too courteous to ask their visitors to leave.

Mallet (1993) and Behi (1992) highlight the benefit of integrating laughter and humour into patient care. Both need to be used cautiously, but when used appropriately, the benefits are great. They may reduce the stress and anxiety felt by patients and staff alike. Humour can also break down barriers between the patient and clinicians, easing embarrassing or awkward situations.

Additionally, humour and laughter can be integrated into patient education, making the presentation of information attractive and easy to understand, such as the *Videos for patients* series by John Cleese on ulcerative colitis
and Crohn's disease.

Admission to hospital and adapting to illness are not pleasant or easy tasks.
It is the responsibility of all nurses to aid the transition as much as possible.

COMPLEMENTARY THERAPIES

Complementary therapies can be attractive to long-term sufferers of
inflammatory bowel disease who have an interest in these therapies and/or
who have experienced insufficient relief from more conventional treatment.
Some therapies which may be considered are:

- dietary restriction/manipulation
- relaxation techniques
- hypnotherapy
- acupuncture
- stress management
- herbal, homoeopathic and naturopathic methods
- aromatherapy.

To some, it would appear obvious that dietary factors may be important in
bowel disorders in view of the logical association, and various regimes
including elemental diets, low residue diets and lactose-free diets have been
found to be helpful, particularly for patients with Crohn's disease (Dowson
1993).

THE SOCIAL CONSEQUENCES OF IBD

It is evident that the symptoms of inflammatory bowel disease are stressful,
and 'have an impact on the ability to function in a variety of roles' (Joachim &
Milne 1985).

Employment

Employment and career prospects are important to maintain self-esteem,
ambition, financial independence and security for personal and family life. A
diagnosis of inflammatory bowel disease may be seen to jeopardise employment prospects and career development. However, it is important to emphasise that most IBD patients live a normal life and only have to take time off
work during exacerbations of inflammation.

Although young people with IBD gain equivalent qualifications to those
without the disease, they often fail to achieve equivalent employment.
Moody et al (1992) addressed this issue of gaining employment and noted
that companies, although denying discrimination, actually fail to employ as
many IBD sufferers as would be expected. Employers are perhaps cautious of
employing sufferers due to fears of cross-infection and loss of working hours
due to ill health and clinic appointments, as well as fear of the unknown. The
current economic climate does not accommodate employees who may not be
cost-effective.

Companies who fail to employ IBD sufferers highlight their lack of knowledge and understanding of the disease. Unfortunately, this attitude has forced individuals to hide their disease by failing to turn up to job interviews or failing to disclose their illness to future employers due to fear of a relapse. Sufferers are forced to modify and adapt their jobs to accommodate the fatigue and malaise they may experience, as well as ensuring hygienic toilet facilities are close by. As a result, promotion prospects and job variation are also affected. This can result in the person becoming demoralised and disillusioned with life.

The attitude of employers is disappointing and inappropriate – in fact, Mayberry & Mayberry (1992) identified that sufferers of Crohn's disease are actually reliable and conscientious workers. Sufferers take very little time off work, resulting in a more impressive attendance record than 'healthy' employees who often fail to turn up to work as a result of minor illnesses and symptoms such as influenza or colds. In addition, IBD sufferers often feel they have to work extremely hard to prove their worth to employers and to compensate for time off sick.

Exercise and sport

Exercise has many benefits for the individual, such as maintaining or gaining fitness, increasing muscle tone and stamina, and increasing the individual's sense of achievement and well-being. Sport and recreational activities are also important in socialisation and team-building. Sufferers of IBD may find they become tired very quickly when partaking in physical activities and exercise. As a result, they may find their hobbies, forms of socialisation and relaxation are reduced or modified. To compound the situation, it is suggested that people who have calcium depletion and/or are on long-term steroid treatment should not partake in contact sports due to the increased risk of fractures. Advice should be sought from the patient's gastroenterologist (Cooke 1991).

Domestic arrangements

During a relapse of ulcerative colitis or Crohn's disease, many clients find domestic chores difficult and tiring. Electrolyte imbalance or anaemia can leave the individual incapable of housework. Shopping, socialising and even collecting the children from school can also become difficult when sufferers are exhausted or needing urgent access to a lavatory (Mallet et al 1978).

Altered body image

Body image can be defined as 'the picture of our own body which we form in our mind, that is to say the way in which our body appears to ourselves' (Schilder 1935). Western society places great importance on having a healthy, slim and sexually desirable body. Failure to achieve this may leave an individual feeling worthless, vulnerable and lacking self-esteem.

The idea of how our body should appear to others is shaped by a number of influences:

- media
- fashion

- culture
- socialisation by parents and teachers
- peers
- employers
- medical personnel
- neurological development
- government health initiatives.

For patients with ulcerative colitis or Crohn's disease, the shape, size and physical appearance of their bodies can change dramatically according to the severity of their disease and its course of treatment. Alterations to the body image can be either permanent or temporary. Consider, for example:

- Incontinence.
- Fistulas.
- Skin tags.
- Surgery, resulting in wounds or scars.
- Stoma formation – in general, stoma formation causes the patient anxiety. Many clients are shocked and feel like freaks when they view their newly formed stomas; females often liken their ileostomies to phallic symbols (see Ch. 4).
- Medication – steroids, although an important part of treatment also carry with them the side-effects of weight gain, mood swings and moon-faced appearance. Although the side effects are generally temporary, they can be quite distressing to the sufferer.
- Fluctuation in weight – due to steroids, malabsorption, diarrhoea or weight gain during periods of remission.
- Nasogastric tube – sometimes used for the administration of elemental diet as patients find it unpleasant to drink.
- Total parenteral nutrition lines – patients' lines may be inserted for a minimum of 2 weeks or more.
- Paediatric problems – Crohn's disease has been shown to stunt growth and sexual development in children. As a result of their disease, children feel different from their peers, miss time from school and are often treated as younger than their years due to their youthful appearance. Consequently, many young adults find it difficult to establish their independence (NACC 1991).
- Sexual dysfunction – clients who have had pelvic surgery for treatment of their IBD may find that their sexual function is disrupted. Additionally, many people suffering from IBD feel uncomfortable and anxious performing sexual activities due to pain or fear of incontinence. Treatment of the disease can also interfere with sexual acts and intimacy; e.g. those who administer enemas are advised to lie on their left side overnight, possibly interfering with their normal sexual or sleeping habits (NACC 1993).

The nurse's role
Some patients do have the opportunity to prepare themselves psychological-

ly and physically for changes to their body. However, a sudden intervention, such as an emergency stoma formation, can have a dramatic impact on an individual's perception of their body. In both situations, the input of nursing staff in certain areas can play a significant role in helping the patient to adapt, as discussed below.

Assessment of fears and worries
Provision of education/support. The patient should be referred to relevant disciplines e.g. stoma therapist and counsellors, and should be provided with information about significant support agencies, such as NACC, Colostomy Association, Ileostomy Association, Relate, and with practical help, i.e. where to get help in an emergency, disposal and acquisition of stoma appliances, tips for travelling, and help with the education of patients and their families regarding their disease, treatment and expected outcomes. Nurses can empower patients by providing information that allows them to become involved in their own care and to make informed decisions about their future and their body.

For those patients who find their medical management failing, surgery is often imminent. At this stage, patients often do not wish to address the consequences of surgery. By virtue of a good therapeutic rapport, the nurse can encourage the patient to address such issues so they can begin to adapt, accept and face up to the implication surgery might have on their lives.

Pre-operative preparation. The nurse can help to foresee any difficulties, and with the siting of the stoma; this latter task should be conducted by an informed stoma therapist (see Ch. 4).

Normalisation. Patients with an altered body image may feel that they are no longer normal. Nurses can help to alleviate this feeling by educating the individual about their disease; treating them as an equal; and introducing the patient to others in a similar situation.

Nurse's reaction. Patients observe nurses' reactions to the sight of their naked body, the smell of their stoma output and their appearance in general. Knowing this, nurses can adapt their responses accordingly. Verbal and non-verbal responses are powerful and can be damaging or uplifting to the vulnerable patient. Verbally, the nurse who adopts a non-critical, positive, but honest attitude is most constructive. Non-verbally, the patient's feelings can be seen to be valued by the use of active listening and touch. Portraying a sense of caring through interactions can instil feelings of importance and respect, and develops a comfortable atmosphere in which to express fears and worries.

Planning and evaluation of care. An individualised, patient-centred focus encourages the client to participate in and influence their care.

Reproduction
Inflammatory bowel disease may begin in early adult life and therefore may coexist, whether active or not, with the reproductive years of many people with IBD (Khosla et al 1984).

Fertility

Both men and women who suffer from inflammatory bowel disease may experience fertility problems.

Women. There is no significant difference between the number of infertile women with a diagnosis of ulcerative colitis and the rest of the population. However, Crohn's disease sufferers are half as likely to become pregnant. Factors suggested for this underlying subfertility are tubal occlusion, nutritional deficiencies and the presence of active disease (Miller 1986). One should also question the frequency of sexual activity as the women may experience dyspareunia due to inflammation in the pelvis.

Men. Male fertility has been shown to be affected by the use of sulphasalazine to maintain disease control. This is temporary and is rapidly reversed on withdrawal of the drug.

Contraception

The oral contraceptive pill has been implicated in the aetiology of Crohn's disease leading to a slightly higher incidence in the women who take it. However, relapse is more frequent in patients with Crohn's disease who continue to take the pill than in those who do not. It is also possible that an oral contraceptive taken by a woman with diarrhoea is less effective and some clinicians would also advise using a barrier method of contraception. Although the 'morning after' pill is absorbed in the small bowel, it should be effective even though absorption is unpredictable, as the dose of oestrogen is extremely high. Other methods of contraception, e.g. intrauterine devices, are not affected by inflammatory bowel disease.

Pregnancy

Women with inflammatory bowel disease are best advised to avoid conception until their disease is inactive, as they may have an increased risk of exacerbating their disease and are then more likely to continue to have symptoms throughout the pregnancy despite medical treatment.

Furthermore, women with active inflammatory bowel disease tend to have higher rates of miscarriages, more complicated pregnancies and lower birthweight babies than women in whom the disease in quiescent (Miller 1986).

If the disease is in remission at the start of the pregnancy, there is a good chance that it will remain in remission throughout the pregnancy and the puerperium. Remission is best maintained by continuing salicylate drugs during pregnancy. There is no reason to suspect that Caesarean sections are more common for Crohn's disease sufferers, (except perhaps where the disease has involved the perineum, cervix and / or the vagina), so a normal vaginal delivery can be expected.

If the pregnant woman experiences an exacerbation (this is most likely to happen in the first trimester), she should be treated in the usual way, as the risks to the mother from active IBD are greater than the risks to the fetus from the treatment (Travis et al 1993).

Assessment of disease activity can be difficult during pregnancy, especially in Crohn's disease, since X-rays must be avoided. Full colonoscopy is also inadvisable but rigid and flexible sigmoidoscopies are safe, although most clinicians avoid these procedures during the first trimester. Magnetic resonance imaging (MRI) has been shown to be very useful in Crohn's disease and is thought to be safe. However, because it has only recently been introduced, there is limited experience and it is generally recommended that it be avoided during the first trimester.

Management of the disease should follow the same principles as for non-pregnant patients. Corticosteroids and sulphasalazine are safe to use during pregnancy – the risk to the pregnancy of uncontrolled mucosal inflammation is greater than the theoretical risks of drug-induced abnormalities. Patients with severe active disease need hospital admission and intravenous steroids. Opinions vary whether azathioprine should be used during pregnancy, but preliminary studies suggest that it is safe and can be used for the control of steroid-dependent disease. However, women are generally advised against conceiving while receiving azathioprine. Finally, surgical resection may be required during pregnancy – the outcome is usually favourable but spontaneous abortion may occur.

Breast-feeding
Sulphasalazine and mesalazine may be passed into breast milk but the amount is very small. Therefore, women taking these and low-dose steroids should be advised that they can breast-feed.

The menopause
Ulcerative colitis is not associated with an early menopause, but Crohn's disease is. Various environmental factors influence the age at menopause and include occupation and smoking habits. Smoking has consistently been shown to be associated with an early menopause and it is linked to Crohn's disease, but the early menopause cannot be attributed solely to smoking habits. The onset of the disease in middle age may also precipitate the menopause (Lichtarowicz et al 1989).

Normal menstruation and the menopause are also related to nutritional status. Nutrition is usually normal in ulcerative colitis, with the exception of severely ill patients. In contrast, patients with Crohn's disease are often poorly nourished in both acute and long-term situations. In Crohn's disease, those with serious nutritional problems can develop amenorrhoea, but may subsequently recommence menstruation with improved nutrition (Lichtarowicz et al 1991).

Adoption
Sadly, adoption agencies do not favour people with chronic illness when they are looking for prospective parents. However, some of the smaller agencies may be more helpful.

Travelling
Some people who suffer from inflammatory bowel disease may be worried about travelling, especially abroad. As long as they prepare for their trip ade-

quately, they should not experience any problems. They need to take out adequate travel insurance, and, if they are travelling in Europe, obtain an E111 form from the post office, which entitles the traveller to free or reduced-cost emergency medical treatment in most European countries.

Before leaving, they should ensure that they have adequate amounts of any prescribed medications and possibly ask their doctor to write a medical summary to take along with them. Once they are away, they naturally need to take more care than most with what they eat and drink, to prevent exacerbating their condition with a bout of 'holiday tummy'.

The European Federation of Crohn's and Ulcerative Colitis Associations (EFCCA) produces a series of leaflets called 'Travelling with IBD' which offer advice for the country of destination, local doctors specialising in inflammatory bowel disease and a translation list of commonly needed words and phrases.

REFERENCES

Behi R 1992 Using humour as therapy in clinical practice. British Journal of Nursing 1(10):484

Bird H, Hassall J 1993 Self administration of drugs. Scutari Press, London

Buswell, C 1993 A chance to say goodbye. Professional Nurse 8(6):406

Cooke D M 1991 Inflammatory bowel disease: primary health care management of ulcerative colitis and Crohn's disease. Nurse Practitioner 16(8):27–30, 35–39

Department of Health 1995 The patients' charter. HMSO, London

Dowson D 1993 The treatment of inflammatory bowel disease by complementary medicine. Complementary Therapies in Medicine 1:139–142

Drossman D A, Leserman J, Li Z, Mitchell M, Zagami E A, Patrick D L 1991 The rating form of IBD patient concerns: a new measure of health status. Psychosomatic Medicine 53:701–712

Jameson H 1992 The ileo-anal pouch – an alternative to a permanent ileostomy. CliniMed (patient information leaflet)

Joachim G, Milne B 1985 The effects of inflammatory bowel disease on lifestyle. Canadian Nurse 81(10):38–40

Kelly M P 1992 Colitis. Tavistock Routledge, London

Khosla R, Willougby C P, Jewell D P 1984 Crohn's disease and pregnancy. Gut 25:52–56

Lichtarowicz A, Norman C, Calcraft B, Morris J S, Rhodes H, Mayberry J 1989 A study of the menopause, smoking and contraception in women with Crohn's disease. Quarterly Journal of Medicine, New Series 72(276):623–631

Lichtarowicz A, Srivastava E, Norman C et al 1991 A study of the menopause in women with ulcerative colitis. Journal of Obstetrics and Gynaecology 11:361–364

Mallett B J, Bingle J, Lennard Jones J E, Gilon E 1978 Living with disease. The Lancet 16:619–621

Mayberry M K, Mayberry J F 1992 Social consequences of inflammatory bowel disease. Hospital Update 18(10):733, 751

Meadows C, Mortensen N, Satsangi J, Snaith R, Storrie J 1994 The ileo-anal pouch. A trouble-shooting guide. John Radcliffe Hospital, Oxford

Miller J P 1986 Inflammatory bowel disease in pregnancy: A review. Journal of The Royal Society of Medicine 79:221–225

Moody G A, Probert C S J, Jayanthi V, Mayberry J F 1992 The attitude of employers to people with inflammatory bowel disease. Social Science and Medicine 34:459–460

NACC 1991 Crohn's disease (patient information leaflet). NACC, London

NACC 1993 Living with inflammatory bowel disease (patient information leaflet). NACC, London

Rhodes J, Mayberry J F 1986 Ulcerative colitis. Medicine International 2:1056–1062
Schilder P 1935 The image and appearance of the human body. Kogan Paul, London
Travis S P L, Taylor R H, Misiewicz J J 1993 Gastroenterology, 2nd edn. Blackwell
    Scientific Publications, Oxford

FURTHER READING

Curry A, Anderson C 1994 Caring for patients with ulcerative colitis and Crohn's
    disease – a guide for nurses. NACC, London

Gillies D A 1982 Nursing management: a systems approach. W B Saunders,
    Philadelphia

Hayward J 1987 Information – a prescription against pain, 3rd edn. RCN, London

Joachim G, Milne N 1987 Inflammatory bowel disease: effects on lifestyle. Journal of
    Advanced Nursing 12:483–487

Kelly M P 1986 The subjective experience of chronic disease: some implications for the
    management of ulcerative colitis: The Journal of Chronic Disease 39(8):653–666

Probert C S J, Mayberry M, Mayberry J F 1992 Education and young people with
    inflammatory bowel disease. Journal of the Royal Society of Health, June: 112–113

Truelove S, Jewell D P 1974 Intensive intravenous regimen for severe attacks of
    ulcerative colitis. The Lancet June 1:1067–1068

Truelove S C, Willoughby C P, Lee E G, Kettlewell M G W 1978 Further experience in
    the treatment of severe attacks of ulcerative colitis. The Lancet November
    18:1086–1088

USEFUL ADDRESSES

National Association for Colitis and Crohn's disease (NACC), 98A London Road,
    St Albans, Herefordshire AL1 1NX

Crohn's in Childhood Research Association (CICRA), 356 West Barnes Lane, London
    KT3 6NB

Kangaroo Club, Stomatherapy Dept, John Radcliffe Hospital, Headley Way,
    Headington, Oxford OX3 9DU

SPOD (The association to aid the sexual and personal relationships of people with a
    disability), 286 Camden Road, London N7 OBJ

National Association for the Childless, 318 Summer Lane, Birmingham, B19 3RL

The British Agency for Adoption and Fostering, 11 Southwark Street, London SE1 1RQ

Relate: local agencies detailed in area telephone directories

Ileostomy Association of Great Britain and Ireland, Amblehurst House, Black Scotch
    Lane, Mansfield NG18 4PF

British Colostomy Association, 38–39 Ecclestone Square, London

European Federation of Crohn's and Ulcerative Colitis Associations, c/o
    Mr J Chandler, 3 Willow Grove, Wellwyn Garden City, Hertfordshire AL8 7NA

Stoma and fistula care

Catherine Meadows

4

■ CONTENTS

Introduction
Surgical construction
Characteristic output of
gastrointestinal stomas
Pre-operative considerations
Postoperative assessement of the
newly formed stoma
First impressions
Common complications

Selecting an appropriate stoma
appliance
Emptying the bag
Performing stoma care
Eating and drinking
Sexual dysfunction related to
stoma surgery
Social support
The enterocutaneous fistula

INTRODUCTION

All nurses in the field of gastroenterology will at some point be involved in the care of a patient with a stoma or an enterocutaneous fistula. As with patients in other areas of care, stoma and fistula patients need nurses who will provide information, support, sensitivity and good communication, but often on a more intimate level. Whilst it is recognised that some may regard the practical 'hands on' management of these patients as less than desirable, their comprehensive care can pose the ultimate nursing challenge. The aim of this chapter is to demystify some aspects of stoma and fistula management, and to provide practical solutions to common problems and information to assist in care planning.

Common conditions which predispose to surgery resulting in stoma formation are:

- ulcerative colitis
- Crohn's disease
- carcinoma
- diverticular disease
- polyposis coli
- ischaemia
- trauma
- radiation damage
- congenital anomalies
- constipation
- incontinence.

Stomas are divided into three types for the purpose of this chapter:

- input or feeding stomas
- output stomas
- diverting or defunctioning stomas.

Input stoma

This is often a temporary measure to facilitate nutrition in patients otherwise unable to take nutrients into the gut. Feeding is via a tube in liquid form, such as a gastrostomy or jejunostomy. Input stomas will not be discussed further in this chapter.

Output stoma

The bowel is brought to the skin surface providing an outlet for body waste.

Diverting or defunctioning stoma

The bowel is brought to the skin surface to divert the flow of body waste away from a diseased segment or a newly formed anastomosis.

SURGICAL CONSTRUCTION

Stomas are commonly formed in one of four ways: end, loop, double-barrelled or split.

End stoma

This is formed by dividing the bowel and bringing up the proximal end as a stoma with a single lumen. The distal bowel is either removed or oversewn and left in the abdominal cavity (see Fig. 4.1).

When the distal bowel including the rectum and anus is removed, the stoma is permanent. This is commonly referred to as an end stoma. For example the Brooke ileostomy is named after the London surgeon who described the technique. The technique was to evert the end of the ileum, exposing the mucosa, and to suture the stoma to the skin (Brooke 1952).

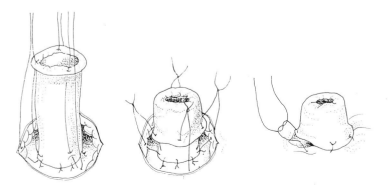

Fig 4.1 Formation of end ileostomy.

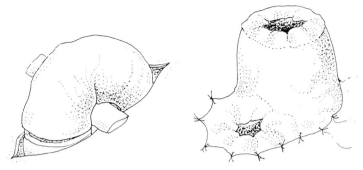

Fig 4.2 Formation of loop ileostomy.

Loop stoma

This is formed by bringing a loop of bowel to the skin surface and then making an incision in the anterior wall to allow faeces to discharge (Fig. 4.2). The resulting stoma has two openings, but the posterior wall separates them. Loop stomas are usually temporary or palliative.

Double-barrelled stoma

This is formed by diverting the bowel and bringing both the proximal and distal ends to the skin surface as two stomas. The two limbs are sutured together side to side. The distal bowel is non-functioning; the proximal end is the functioning or output stoma. The double-barrelled stoma is usually temporary or palliative.

Split stoma

This is formed when the proximal and distal segments of bowel are brought to the skin surface some distance apart, e.g. one in the right iliac fossa and one in the left iliac fossa. The distal segment stoma is known as a mucous fistula.

Ileostomy

Indications for loop ileostomy

- To defunction the distal bowel after resection, thereby protecting the anastomosis, e.g. anterior resection, ileal pouch anal anastomosis (see Fig. 4.3 E and F). The ileostomy will be reversed after approximately 8–12 weeks, providing the anastomosis is viable.
- To "rest" diseased bowel with the aim of alleviating symptoms, e.g. Crohn's disease.
- To provide proximal diversion in cases of obstruction or fistula, e.g. obstructing carcinoma, rectovaginal fistula.

Usual site. Right iliac fossa.

Indications for end ileostomy

- Where the entire colon, rectum and anus must be removed, resulting in a permanent ileostomy, e.g. Crohn's colitis, ulcerative colitis, familial adenomatous polyposis (see Fig. 4.3 B). This operation is known as a panproctocolectomy. With current advances in surgical techniques, permanent ileostomy is less common, because most patients with ulcerative colitis and familial adenomatous polyposis will be offered an ileal pouch anal anastomosis.

- Occasionally, where there is a loss of colonic motility or failure of pelvic floor mechanism causing chronic constipation.

Usual site.   Right iliac fossa.

Indication for double-barrelled and split ileostomy
- When complete diversion of the faecal flow is necessary, e.g. Crohn's disease. The mucous fistula can act as an input stoma for steroid enemas.

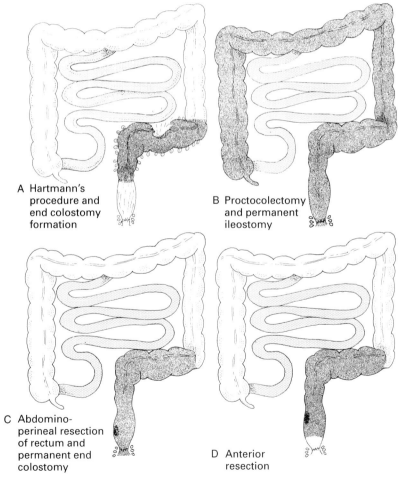

A Hartmann's procedure and end colostomy formation

B Proctocolectomy and permanent ileostomy

C Abdomino-perineal resection of rectum and permanent end colostomy

D Anterior resection

Fig 4.3 Bowel resections: shaded area represents length of gut resected.

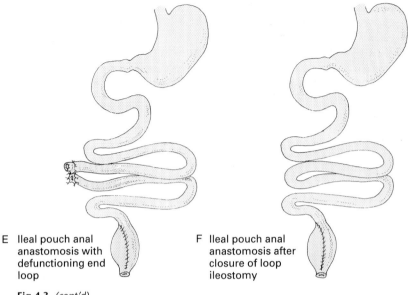

E Ileal pouch anal
   anastomosis with
   defunctioning end
   loop

F Ileal pouch anal
   anastomosis after
   closure of loop
   ileostomy

Fig 4.3 *(cont'd)*

- When the viability of both segments of bowel need to be monitored, e.g. after resection of a necrotic segment.

Usual site. Right iliac fossa with the mucous fistula above or on the other side of the abdomen.

Colostomy

Indications for loop colostomy

- To defunction distal bowel where there is an obstructing lesion. This may be an interim measure during which time the patient receives radiotherapy to render the lesion operable at a later date. Loop colostomy may also be a palliative measure where no further treatment will be given but the symptoms of obstruction will be alleviated. Sigmoid or transverse colon is usually used.
- To defunction distal bowel after resection to protect the anastomosis. The colostomy will usually be reversed after a period of approximately 8–12 weeks, providing the anastomosis is viable.
- To defunction the bowel to alleviate the symptoms of radiation enteritis.
- To provide a faecal diversion in the presence of a rectovaginal fistula or colovesical fistula, or after repair of the above. The length of time that the stoma is present will be determined by the healing of the fistula or the anastomosis.

Usual site. Transverse loop colostomy – right upper quadrant; sigmoid loop colostomy – left iliac fossa.

Indications for end colostomy
* Where it is necessary to remove the rectum and anus, e.g. abdominoperineal excision of rectum for carcinoma (see Fig. 4.3 C)
* Where it is necessary to completely transect the descending or sigmoid colon to defunction the distal segment of bowel, e.g. Hartmann's procedure (see Fig. 4.3 A) for perforated sigmoid colon or diverticular abscess (Cuschieri et al 1988)
* End colostomy is less common but may be successfully formed to alleviate the embarrassing symptoms of incontinence. The distal bowel is usually left inside the abdominal cavity.

Usual site. Left iliac fossa.

Caecostomy
This is rarely performed these days, but caecostomy is a means of decompressing the colon in an emergency. The fluid output from the caecum together with the skin-flush stoma are potentially problematic in terms of skin care.

For temporary decompression of the colon, a caecostomy tube may be inserted. After the easy removal procedure, there is no need for further surgery to close the stoma.

CHARACTERISTIC OUTPUT OF GASTROINTESTINAL STOMAS

Various factors may influence the characteristics of the output of each stoma, e.g. diet, medication, amount of bowel resected. As a general rule, the more proximal the stoma, the more fluid is the effluent, and the more caustic its effect on the skin due to the presence of proteolytic enzymes (see Table 4.1).

The skin is naturally slightly acidic, and therefore effluent that is very slightly acidic or neutral is less likely to cause skin damage. Effluent that is markedly acidic or alkaline will be more damaging to the skin. However, high volumes of liquid effluent can cause maceration where peristomal skin is inadequately protected, whether or not it is naturally caustic. This is usually due to pooling of the effluent in the peristomal area.

Table 4.1 Characteristic output of stoma

Type of Stoma	Volume/24 h (m/s)	Consistency
Jejunostomy	1000–3000	Liquid
Ileostomy	500–1000	Porridge
Caecostomy/ascending colostomy	500–750	Porridge
Transverse colostomy		Semi-formed
Descending/sigmoid colostomy		Semi-formed to formed

PRE-OPERATIVE CONSIDERATIONS

Assessing the prospective patient

Before the nursing team can plan the care of a prospective ostomist, the patient's needs must be determined. These needs can be based on an initial assessment of his status, resources and social support. Pre-operative preparation may begin weeks or even months before the planned surgery and may include visits to the stomatherapy nurse, the surgeon or the general practitioner. By the time the patient arrives on the surgical ward, he may have been afforded the luxury of time to absorb and make sense of the information he has been given. However, if this is not the case, the pre-operative assessment will be carried out 1 or 2 days prior to surgery.

The aims of the pre-operative assessment are:

- To determine the patient's ability to cope with a stoma on a practical basis
- To gain insight into the features of the patient's usual style of living and to estimate his ability to return to this level after surgery
- To identify any compromises or modifications that the patient may have to consider for his rehabilitation.

Eyesight

Planning the care and teaching of a visually impaired patient involves careful selection of site, stoma equipment and a creative and flexible nursing team. Stoma care for the blind or visually impaired is often performed by touch. If the patient normally wears spectacles, they should be questioned as to whether they are suitable for looking straight down towards the abdomen. Bifocals, for instance, may not provide the necessary magnification when looking sharply downwards. The visually impaired patient sometimes finds it easier to perform stoma care in a mirror, possibly with magnification. Models for the patient to practise on may be helpful. Audio tapes with information and instruction may provide further assistance.

Manual dexterity

Does the patient have compromised dexterity? For example, does she suffer from arthritis, or has she had a stroke? The limit of the patient's ability may be easily assessed by asking such questions as: 'can you do up buttons?'; 'can you tie shoelaces?'; 'do you knit, write, or sew?'

Individual selection of an appliance by testing the patient with each type may be time-consuming, but it will ensure that the best possible option is taken. The patient can practise clamping and releasing on an empty stoma bag or practise placing and securing the chosen appliance to a model or another area of her body.

It is fortunate that, in the UK, there is a wide selection of stoma appliances available to choose from. The health care team will understand that they may need to give the patient more time than most require for postoperative recovery to become well practised in stoma care. It is essential that the patient has confidence in her ability before discharge.

Mental/emotional state

Kelly (1992) states that 'a doctor's recommendation for surgery does not result in automatic acceptance and compliance', especially for a procedure such as stoma surgery. To fully realise the implications of stoma surgery, the patient needs to be capable of applying the given information to herself and her individual situation. Deliberate and direct questioning may be necessary to ascertain the patient's feelings and perceived ideas about the operation, so that any misconceptions may be rectified. Patients often have a very negative view of life with a stoma if they know somebody else who has had the same operation and who is not doing very well.

Distress and/or anxiety among the spouse and family will affect the patient and therefore it is important to give other family members the opportunity to express their feelings about the illness and the operation. In so doing, the patient may be indirectly treated.

Anxiety about the diagnosis may be a significant factor affecting the emotional state of patients awaiting stoma surgery, especially considering that one of the main conditions predisposing to stoma formation is cancer. Identifying specific problems and sharing concerns may help the patient to cope with the situation. Acknowledgement that her fears are justified will make it easier for her to address and discuss them.

Sharing concerns with somebody who has had a similar experience can often provide encouragement. Acknowledging the seriousness of the operation and comparing notes with that person about feelings towards the prospect of having a stoma may offer 'impartial' information and empathy. Most stomatherapy nurses will have a list of people who are willing to 'visit' new ostomists.

Cultural considerations

Acknowledging cultural differences is imperative in the management of care of the prospective stoma patient.

Language barriers may pose difficulties during information giving, but finding a suitable interpreter may not be as easy as it might at first seem. For example, it may be highly inappropriate in some cultures for a male member of the family to discuss the toileting habits or the problems of vaginal discharge with a female member. This may be the case even in married couples. For example, when introducing the fact that during abdominoperineal excision of the rectum, the posterior vaginal wall may be excised, the interpreter/husband may not pass on this information to his wife.

The cultural and religious needs of each individual must be addressed properly and potential problems anticipated. For example, people who perform a prayer ritual or prostration will have specific needs in terms of the choice of appliance. They will need to know that the appliance will be secure during these important activities. By addressing the future as well as the immediate pre- and postoperative period, misapprehensions may be avoided.

Choosing a site for the stoma

Crucial to the successful outcome of stoma formation is the selection of the site. This should ideally be done by somebody well-practised in the procedure and who can devote as much time as the patient needs during selection, e.g. a stomatherapy nurse.

Factors to consider

The rectus muscle
To minimise the risk of the stoma prolapsing, it may be sited within the rectus muscle (vertical sheet of muscle between the diaphragm and the pubis). The muscle can be identified by palpation and the width ascertained.

Skin folds
Bulges, rolls and folds of skin can cause problems for the patient with a stoma. A flat skin area in the required quadrant of the abdomen is desirable. Time should be devoted to assessing the surface anatomy and body contours, with the patient changing position periodically. The potential site should be marked with an indelible pen and the patient then asked to change position to assess the appropriateness. About 6–7 cm square of flat skin is ideal for the adhesion of a flange or one-piece bag.

Other considerations
Scars, bony prominences, the umbilicus and the patient's belt or waistline should be avoided if at all possible. The patient's usual style of dress is important to consider and it may be appropriate to ask them to bring into hospital any particular garment that they may have concerns about, e.g. a swimsuit with a high cut leg. The need for supportive garments, e.g. corset or back support, may be a complicating factor during stoma siting, but they must nevertheless be included in the assessment.

The visibility of the stoma by the patient may make the difference between achieving independent self-care or not. Whilst the use of mirrors to perform stoma care is acceptable, being able to see the stoma easily on the abdomen may give the patient more confidence in her ability. Sporting activities and hobbies will need to be taken into consideration, e.g. supportive or protective clothing may pose difficulties.

If time allows, the patient may wish to wear a stoma bag for a few hours prior to surgery so that the chosen position may be assessed.

In cases of very poorly sited stomas, the worst-case scenario would be re-operation. Hence, it should be a professional who is well-practised in stoma care who guides patients through the siting procedure and helps them to choose a suitable position. It is imperative that the patient understands that all aspects of her life can be addressed and discussed.

The patient's attitude towards surgery should be elicited and any preconceived ideas about living with a stoma should be discussed. At this point, any 'old wives' tales' ('can't bath or swim'; 'you'll be housebound'; 'you'll have to register disabled', etc.) should be addressed or dispelled. Positive attitudes should be reinforced.

The use of a nursing model, such as the Roy Adaptation Model (Roy 1984) to assess the patient may ensure that all needs and potential problems are addressed. Roy's model is explained in Chapter 7.

The following components of the patient's lifestyle need to be explored in relation to the stoma and any adjustments that may be required can be discussed:

1. Self–concept
   — who knows about the operation and its implications?
   — sexual activity: is this threatened?
   — general demeanour
   — level of education
   — heterosexual or homosexual?

2. Role function
   — dependants/marital status/significant others?
   — does the patient need help to explain the operation to them?
   — sleeping arrangements
   — occupation
   — returning to work/unemployment
   — contraception.

3. Interdependence
   — who lives at home?
   — bathroom facilities
   — social life/hobbies/travel/sport
   — financial worries
   — employer support.

4. Physiological
   — special diet
   — eating patterns
   — favourite foods
   — medication/allergies
   — skin condition
   — social life/sport
   — stature/general health.

Providing information about forthcoming surgery

The ability of the patient to apply the information to himself and his lifestyle will depend on his understanding of the impending surgery.

A review of studies by Corney (1991) indicates that most patients wish to know as much as possible about their illness, its causes, treatment and outcome. Studies of a range of surgical patients show generally positive results from giving adequate information and preparation before surgery and also show that preparation can affect postoperative pain and the time taken to recover as well as anxiety levels. For the prospective stoma patient, the benefits of pre-operative information and preparation are more obvious, as there is often an overwhelming amount of information that would be very difficult to assimilate whilst recovering from a general anaesthetic. This highlights the plight of the patient who receives emergency surgery, in which case the ability of the patient to cope with technical details and descriptions needs careful consideration. If it is possible that the patient may require stoma formation during emergency surgery, then, if time and the situation allow, a suitable position for the stoma should be marked on his body. However, if he is very distended, this may be impossible to perform effectively. A brief explanation of the possibility that a stoma may be required is important, as is giving the patient the option to seek further information if he feels he can deal with it at that time. Often, a very brief description of the function and practical management of a stoma can serve to allay fears about radical body changes and a ruined lifestyle.

Whilst levels of intelligence differ, and some patients will seek as much information as possible, a basic explanation of the anatomy of the gut and the mechanics of the surgery should be given. The use of simple diagrams may make it easier for the patient to understand and may also make it easier for the nurse to explain. Many patients, for instance, might not realise that whilst stool is being expelled from the stoma in the abdomen, the distal gut may still be in place and may produce 'a discharge'. In this case, a diagram showing a defunctioning loop stoma would be a useful aid, showing the direction of the flow of stool and an explanation of the function of gut mucosa.

Photographs together with a description of the stoma will give patients a better idea of how their abdomen will look after the operation. Useful adjectives include 'moist', 'red' and 'pink'. The spout of an ileostomy should always be explained as it may be a shock postoperatively, especially to women, who often describe the appearance as 'like a penis' – 'similar to the inside of one's cheek or lower lip' is a good description. Bowel muscle action should be described so that the natural visible contraction of the bowel is an anticipated sight and not a horrific one.

POSTOPERATIVE ASSESSMENT OF THE NEWLY FORMED STOMA

Postoperative assessment and documentation are imperative for the evaluation of the patient's well-being and status in relation to a speedy recovery. Documented evaluation should be easy to interpret by members of the health care team and should provide them with a baseline for assessment, especially in the event of a change in the patient's condition.

The initial baseline assessment should include the following characteristics of the stoma:

- stoma type
- colour
- size
- location
- length.

Stoma type

It it a loop or an end stoma? Which part of the bowel has been brought to the surface? If there is more than one stoma, e.g. there is the presence of a mucous fistula, then identify which stoma is proximal and which is distal.

Colour

Ideally, stomas should be red and moist. Any dark or dusky areas should be documented and reported to the stomatherapist or the medical staff.

Size

An approximate size should be ascertained if the stoma bag is intact. Measurement in mm is generally used in stoma care – this will give colleagues some idea about the size of the appliance to be used after the 'post-op' bag is removed.

Length

This is important in establishing the degree of difficulty that the patient is likely to have when commencing self-care and also in monitoring for prolapse. Stoma length can change when the patient begins to recover mobility postoperatively and begins to use her abdominal muscles.

Location

Where on the abdomen is the stoma situated? Proximity to wounds, drain sites, etc. is worth noting and any difficulties the patient may have should be anticipated when he begins self-care – e.g. will he have to work around a suprapubic catheter?

Day-to-day assessement

While documentation of the length, size and colour remains important, examination of the peristomal area in general should also include the following.

Mucocutaneous junction

The mucocutaneous junction is the site at which the mucosa of the bowel joins the skin. Sutures around the stoma are usually dissolvable but the presence of any that may need removing should be noted as these may be 'forgotten'. Any separation at the mucocutaneous junction should be documented by using the numbers of a clock face to describe the location, with 12 o'clock in line with the patient's head, e.g. 'small areas of mucocutaneous separation noted at 3–4 o'clock'.

Peristomal skin condition

Any redness, inflammation or broken areas must be noted as these may indicate a problem with the management of the stoma. The cause of the skin reaction should be investigated immediately.

Surface anatomy of peristomal area

The presence of creases, recession of the stoma into an indentation, and the position of the stoma in relation to skin folds or bulges should be noted.

The ideal stoma is red and moist and protrudes approximately 20 mm from the skin surface. This protrusion facilitates drainage of the effluent away from the peristomal skin and into the stoma bag. However, colostomies are often relatively flush with the skin. Skin-flush stomas may be more difficult to manage in cases of liquid output. However, a stoma that is excessively long may be equally difficult for the patient to manage when applying a bag; is more susceptible to damage; and may be visible as a bulge under clothing.

A round stoma is easier to accommodate in terms of fitting appliances, as cutting guides are usually designed with concentric circles. Appliances are manufactured in pre-cut round shapes. The patient may, however, cut her own appliance to fit, or may enlist the help of certain commercial organisations who offer this service. The lumen or stomal orifice is best situated at the apex of the stoma to facilitate drainage of effluent into the bag and not divert it towards the skin surface.

A flat, crease-free area of skin that is both below the waistline and visible to the patient is obviously preferable to one that is located near bony prominences, skin folds and scars. This will optimise the chances of a well-sealed appliance, which is easier to conceal under clothes.

FIRST IMPRESSIONS

The patient's first impression will be a long-lasting one. Sensitivity, competence and discretion are therefore extremely important when teaching a new stoma patient how to change the bag. When the bag is removed for the first time, the patient very often watches the expression on the nurses's face rather than the stoma. Reassuring glances and a calm and confident manner may prevent feelings of revulsion and abnormality.

Sitting by the side of the patient during stoma care teaching is beneficial for both patient and nurse. Giving the patient the impression that there is plenty of time may encourage her to ask questions or raise issues that may be troubling her. Standing and bending over the patient, apart from being uncomfortable, may give the impression that there is not much time and also that the nurse does not wish to be close to the patient.

A description of the stoma whilst handling it is useful – say, for example, 'this is a nice healthy looking ileostomy. It's red and moist and has a small spout, which is good. At the moment it's a bit swollen but it will reduce in size over the next few weeks. Did you notice that there is no sensitivity in the ileostomy? You won't feel hot or cold or pain in it, that's normal. You may notice the bowel moving at times – that's just natural muscle contraction and relaxation.'

Acknowledging the fact that there may be a presence of odour should not make the patient feel uncomfortable, but should reassure her that this is usual during bag changes. Ignoring odour or telling the patient that there is no odour may only serve to foster mistrust in the nurses and possibly the fear that she should expect to be smelling whilst she has a stoma.

Patients react in different ways to the odour produced whilst changing a stoma bag. This may depend on past experiences – for example, the odour produced by ileostomy effluent may not be nearly as unpleasant as the odour from the bloody, slimy faeces produced by the patient who has active ulcerative colitis.

These days, gloves should be worn whilst performing any duty that involves contact with body fluids. In years gone by, handling with gloves was assumed to foster feelings of being unclean, leading to a negative reaction to the stoma. However, a simple explanation will ensure that the patient realises that it is for her own protection as well as others'. For example, 'I'm going to wear gloves to change your bag. This is to protect you and others from cross-infection. There is no need for *you* to wear gloves when dealing with your stoma.'

Help the patient to find a comfortable position so that she can see the stoma. Ensuring privacy and lack of disturbance by other staff, sitting down and having time to talk during bag changing will be rewarding, as patients often find these intimate moments appropriate for discussing particular anxieties regarding the stoma. If the patient does not grab the opportunity, it may be appropriate for the nurse to do so. Direct but sensitive questioning regarding the patient's true feelings about the stoma and its implications may be appropriate.

COMMON COMPLICATIONS

Sensitivity to appliance (possible allergy)

Inflamed or broken skin in the peristomal area will compromise the adhesion and therefore the security of the stoma bag, as well as causing discomfort. Most appliance manufacturers today produce hypoallergenic materials, however sensitivity and allergy are not infrequent. Patients with a history of sensitivity to materials or adhesives should be carefully assessed pre-operatively if the situation allows. Testing the patient for sensitivity to stoma appliance materials involves sticking small, carefully labelled patches of each product on another area of the body and monitoring their response over 2 days if possible. The patient may complain of itching, burning or soreness under the appliance.

A sensitivity reaction to the stoma bag or its skin barrier can be identified by removing the appliance and comparing the distribution of the inflamed area with the size and shape of the appliance. The stomatherapy nurse should be informed.

The medical team should be informed if the reaction is severe, painful or extensive, and pharmacological treatment may be necessary.

For patients with intractable problems of sensitivity, a referral to a dermatologist is indicated so that the allergen can be identified.

Herniation

Most commonly seen in patients with end colostomies, parastomal herniation occurs in about 20–25% of cases (Devlin 1982). Sometimes described as resembling a 'breast', the appearance of the hernia can be very distressing. Apart from the bulge being unsightly and sometimes difficult to conceal, anxieties about the return of a tumour may be induced. The patient's usual appliance may be unsuitable; in fact mild or gradual onset of parastomal herniation may be brought to the patient's attention by the stomatherapy nurse investigating the cause of a leaky appliance.

Before treatment is recommended, the patient should be examined by a doctor to confirm the diagnosis and to rule out the possibility of intestinal obstruction due to kinked bowel. Obstruction in a parastomal hernia is recognised by a colicky abdominal pain.

Treatment may be in the form of a support garment in cases of slight herniation. For more marked hernias, surgical revision may be indicated. The stomatherapy nurse may advise the patient regarding abdominal exercises.

Mechanical trauma

Red, painful areas that bleed upon removing the skin barrier around the stoma are usually an indication of trauma caused by stripping of the skin. Common causes are harsh or abrasive cleansing agents, careless removal of the appliance, or an ill-fitting appliance causing friction. Bleeding will compromise adhesion. Simple assessment of the patient's stoma care technique may reveal the cause of mechanical trauma.

Bleeding

Spotting of blood during cleaning is not abnormal and is due to the very vascular mucosa. However, the source of the bleed should be established, as the implications for treatment and consequences are markedly different. Bleeding from the lumen may indicate a serious condition such as an exacerbation of the inflammatory bowel disease, carcinoma or portal hypertension. Bleeding from the mucocutaneous junction, however, may be easily remedied. Common causes of bleeding from the stoma above skin level are:

- trauma – stoma bags that are improperly sized or improperly applied may injure the mucosa, leading to bleeding (Alterescu 1985)
- granuloma – a granuloma may be treated with silver nitrate which gradually 'burns off' the over-granulated layers; a large granuloma may require surgical removal if stoma management becomes a problem.

Prolapse

This is a condition in which the bowel 'telescopes' out from the opening in the skin so that it is longer. This is most commonly seen in transverse loop colostomies and the distal bowel is usually affected, although both limbs of the loop may prolapse (Goligher 1984).

Reassurance that the prolapse is not serious may help to alleviate some of the patient's anxieties, together with support and encouragement and instruction in managing a bigger appliance.

The appearance of prolapsed bowel can be extremely distressing and it can make the stoma very difficult to manage. The stoma will be prone to trauma and may become oedematous or necrosed if constricted.

Vaseline gel applied thickly to the prolapsed bowel may reduce the chances of trauma due to friction. The patient should be made aware of the signs of intestinal obstruction and should observe for colour changes and report them immediately. Surgical repair of a prolapse may be indicated if it is not possible for the patient to manage.

Retraction

This is a condition in which the bowel recedes from the skin. A retracted stoma poses management problems, especially if the effluent is loose, e.g. ileostomy. Possible causes are:

- poor surgical technique – too much tension on the suture line.
- weight gain causing tension
- premature removal of the support rod
- mucocutaneous separation due to infection or necrosis.

Postoperative retraction should receive immediate attention as it may require surgical repair. Even the most established ostomist will need some help in learning to manage the retracted stoma. The use of an appliance with convexity (to encourage the stoma to protrude) and / or a support belt may provide the necessary solution. Weight loss may remedy the situation in the obese patient. Surgical revision may also be indicated if the retraction is considerable and unmanageable.

Ischaemia/necrosis

Observation of the stoma in the early postoperative period is particularly important as this is the most likely time for necrosis to occur. Impaired blood supply to the stoma will cause a purple dusky colour and ischaemia may follow on to necrosis, which would present as black odorous bowel.

Ischaemia and necrosis in the initial postoperative period are usually due to a fault in surgical construction; however, a tight fitting appliance or pressure from very tight-fitting clothes may be the cause in established ostomists. Necrosis requires urgent surgical assessment.

Stenosis

This is a condition where the lumen of the stoma becomes narrowed at either the fascial or cutaneous level. In severe cases, the stoma may close completely. The cause of stenosis in the early postoperative period may be due to surgical technique or mucocutaneous separation. Established colostomists presenting with stenosis may report pain on passing stool and the stools are typically 'ribbon-like'. Ileostomists may present with partial obstruction due to a food blockage.

Treatment with dilators or digital dilatation may prove effective in opening up the lumen, but care must be taken not to split the skin which would cause further scarring. Recognition of the fact that some patients will be unable to insert a dilator or finger into their bodies is important and may prove to be a very sensitive issue. In severe cases, where the patient is having extreme difficulty in passing stools and / or the peristomal skin is affected, surgical revision is indicated.

High-output stoma

The team needs to address the fluid and electrolyte balance of the patient with a high-output stoma. Oral rehydration solutions such as Dioralyte or the World Health Organization solution may be indicated, together with antidiarrhoeal medication such as loperamide. Antidiarrhoeal medication is best taken an hour before eating for maximum effect. The patient should be advised to add salt to their meals if they do not usually.

The stoma is best managed with a system that allows continuous drainage, such as a urostomy appliance or the purpose-designed 'High Output system' (Convatec). Extra skin protection may be indicated, such as Stomahesive Paste (Convatec). Careful monitoring of the general status of the patient is important to detect signs of salt depletion and dehydration.

Admission to hospital for intravenous fluid replacement may be necessary. Oral rehydration solution should be used as a temporary measure.

SELECTING AN APPROPRIATE STOMA APPLIANCE

When selecting the appliance for new patients, the following should be considered:

- the size, shape and degree of protrusion of the stoma
- type and consistency of the effluent
- the body contours of the patient
- the manual dexterity and visual acuity of the patient
- the patient's lifestyle in terms of physical activity
- the patient's preferences regarding shape and colour.

The new stoma patient will usually not have the knowledge to make decisions regarding the type of appliance that is best for her. During the postoperative period, the patient will be guided by the nursing staff. However, once well-practised in caring for the stoma, and when her knowledge has increased, the patient will be able to select her appliance from the range available on the market.

The main deciding factors influencing the patient's choice of stoma appliance will usually be:

- security
- comfort
- discretion.

Aims
- To protect the stoma and the peristomal skin from mechanical trauma
- To protect the peristomal skin from chemical trauma caused by stomal effluent and by the products used in stoma care
- To keep the patient odour-free
- To promote feelings of confidence and security in the patient.

Products available
In the UK there is a wide range of products available. Generally, they are classified as those most suitable for faecal effluent and those most suitable for urine. However, it is often the consistency of the effluent that is influential when deciding which is most appropriate, e.g. jejunostomy effluent which is faecal, is often managed with a urostomy appliance. This is due to the watery consistency of the effluent.

Stoma bags are either drainable or closed (Fig. 4.4).

Drainable bags are open-ended to facilitate the removal of liquid faeces and are secured at the bottom with a plastic clamp or wire tie.

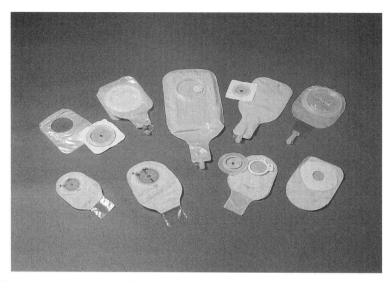

Fig 4.4 A selection of stoma bags and wound managers.

Closed-end bags have no drainage facility and are removed when full. They are most suitable for patients who pass a formed stool.

Urostomy bags are drainable but they also have a non-return film to minimise the flow-back of urine to the stoma and to reduce the chances of excoriation by pooled urine. Urostomy bags also have a tap at the bottom to facilitate easy emptying and to allow an overnight drainage appliance to be attached.

One-piece bags come with a skin-protecting wafer and bag all in one. They may be cut to fit individual stomas or they may come in pre-cut sizes which are round. A one-piece bag has a slim profile and is usually very flexible. Its simplicity is often the reason people choose to use it.

Two-piece bags come with a separate base plate and bag. The base plates come in both cut-to-fit and pre-cut sizes which are round. The two-piece is less slim in profile than the one-piece bag and may be less flexible. However, the two-piece is often chosen for its durability, good visibility when positioning over the stoma (there is no bag in the way), and because patients may change the bag without disturbing the peristomal area.

Re-usable bags are no longer promoted by stoma appliance manufacturers, although they are still available for long-time users. They are made of heavy materials such as rubber and usually require adhesives, skin protectors and belts for security.

The skin barriers and base plates are all manufactured with hypoallergenic materials to minimise the changes of peristomal skin irritation. They can be placed directly onto the skin so that no additional preparation is needed. However, there are accessory products available for the less straightforward stoma.

Commonly used accessory products

Skin barriers. These come in the form of sprays, wipes, gels, roll-ons and liquid. They provide a protective layer when dry for reducing mechanical trauma by repeated removal of the base plate or one-piece appliance. They contain alcohol and will therefore sting on inflamed or broken skin.

Protective wafers. These are usually hypoallergenic materials and come in squares, rings or strips. They are for extra skin protection when necessary.

Powders. Used to absorb moisture on excoriated areas so that the appliance will adhere. Calamine lotion is an alternative. Neither of these products contains alcohol and they are not usually painful on application.

Filler paste. This is made from the same constituents as the skin protectors but often contains alcohol. The paste can be used to fill in creases or indentations to produce a flat area for the base plate to sit on. It is also used as an extra sealant around the stoma when necessary. The paste is usually removed with the skin-protecting wafer or base plate (see Case histories 4.1 and 4.2).

Solvents. These are manufactured specifically for facilitating the removal of stoma care products by breaking the adhesives. The skin should be rinsed after use.

Deodorisers. These come in the form of oils and sprays and have specific uses. Oils are usually dropped into the stoma bag before application to help reduce the odour from faeces on removing the bag. Sprays are either squirted into the bag before applications or used to deodorise the bathroom after the bag has been emptied or changed.

Filters. These are small stick-on charcoal pads; patients can attach a filter to the top of the stoma bag, making a small puncture through into the bag. Flatus is forced out through the small hole in the charcoal and is deodorised as it is expelled. Closed-end bags usually have built-in flatus filters. They are optional for drainable bags (although some are built in). Generally, the filter is more effective when the effluent is of a thicker consistency. The filter should be covered when bathing or swimming to prevent saturation. However, if a vacuum occurs, the stool may stick at the top of the bag. In this situation, the filter should be covered to allow some flatus to release the stool.

EMPTYING THE BAG

This is quite individual. Patients will find the method which best suits them.

Guidelines
The following procedure may be used: sit on the toilet at the back of the seat; open legs; remove clamp from bag whilst holding tail of bag up; turn tail of bag inside out and pour stool into toilet; wipe tail with tissue; unfold tail; reapply clamp.

The emptying may be done while kneeling or standing, or the stool may be placed into a container first, which is then emptied into the toilet. The method used will be determined by the patient's capabilities and preference.

Close-end bags are removed and, if possible, the contents squeezed from the bag into the toilet. Some people keep scissors in the bathroom and cut the top of the bag off to empty the contents. Stoma bags can be disposed of in 'nappy bags', carrier bags, newspaper or other wrapping and then placed in the usual domestic rubbish bin.

PERFORMING STOMA CARE

This is usually a routine which takes place in the patient's toilet or bathroom, as this is the normal place for dealing with elimination and privacy can be ensured.

For the patient who is learning to care for his stoma, the bedside is often the place where he will get his first experience of seeing the stoma and watching the bag being changed.

A snug-fitting appliance will ensure that the peristomal skin is protected; however, if the appliance is too tight around the stoma, leakage, friction and bleeding may occur. A measuring guide will provide assistance when determining the correct size. Approximately 1 mm larger than the actual diameter of the stoma is acceptable. If too much skin is exposed, excoriation, leaking and bleeding may occur.

Procedure

The following procedure is normal practice:

- Organise all equipment that is to be used. You may need:
  — a clean stoma bag cut to fit the stoma, and a clamp if necessary
  — warm water
  — wipes or tissues
  — disposal sack or 'nappy bag'
  — any accessories that may be needed, e.g. solvent.
- Remove the existing bag by peeling downwards whilst supporting the skin with the other hand. Peeling down from top to bottom will ensure that any stool expelled will be collected as it runs down.
- Place the soiled bag in the disposal sack, retaining the clamp if it is a drainable bag.
- Use a dry wipe to pick up the stool and mucus that may be on the stoma and surrounding skin.
- Clean the peristomal area with moist wipes removing any traces of stool or adhesive.
- Dry the peristomal area by patting with a tissue.
- Remove the backing paper from the clean bag and position over the stoma; fold the skin protector over so that the bottom edge of the cut hole can be placed in position under the stoma. The skin protector can then be lifted up and over the stoma and smoothed down.
- Apply the clamp to the bottom of the bag if necessary.
- Dispose of the rubbish appropriately. A template should be left with the patient.

Making a template

Measure or estimate the diameter of the stoma. Cut a circle or a semi-circle in a designated piece of card. Match the size and shape to the stoma and make the necessary adjustments.

Use the template during bag changes to accurately size the aperture of the appliance. During the immediate postoperative period, the stoma may increase in size due to oedema but will eventually reduce. The template will need adjusting accordingly.

Stoma measuring guides are usually provided by appliance manufacturers.

Case history 4.1 Mucocutaneous separation in a patient taking high-dose steroids for Crohn's disease (Fig. 4.5)

The patient presented with persistent leaks from his two-piece system flange. The area was irrigated with saline and dried as much as possible. Calcium alginate fibre was placed firmly into the moist shallow peristomal cavity. Stomahesive paste was added in a thin covering layer. The patient's usual flange was applied but included an insert to produce convexity and improve the seal around the stoma. A drainable bag was added. The patient repeated this procedure every 3 days. The skin was healed after 4 weeks.

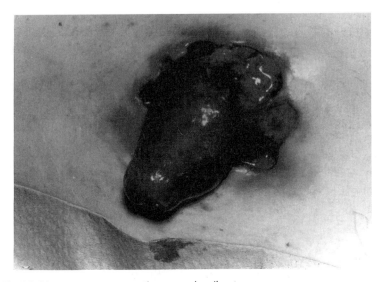

Fig 4.5 Mococutaneous separation around an ileostomy.

EATING AND DRINKING

Generally, a balanced diet and adequate fluid intake must be emphasised. However, there are certain food types that are known to affect stomal output (see Table 4.2).

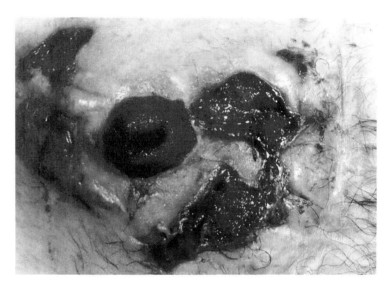

Fig 4.6 Hidradenitis suppuritiva.

Case history 4.2 Hidradenitis suppurativa in a patient with an ileostomy for ulcerative colitis (see Fig. 4.6)

The patient was referred by his GP with a long history of leaking flanges. The skin was irrigated with saline as it was very painful. After careful drying, Granuflex Paste (Convatec) was applied to the moist painful areas. Stomahesive paste was added to encircle the stoma where the skin was unaffected. A hydrocolloid flange was applied followed by a drainable bag. Pain reduction was considerable at the next flange change, and bleeding caused by trauma stopped. Antibiotics were prescribed concurrently. The patient had a secure appliance for the duration of antibiotic therapy. The flange was changed every 3 days.

Control of flatus

Much of the flatus passed from the stoma has been ingested. Ingested air affects the small bowel more than the colon, where it is usually absorbed during transit. Ingested air can be reduced by avoiding chewing gum, smoking, talking while eating and chewing with an open mouth, and by avoiding the use of drinking straws. Flatus is also produced by the bacterial action of undigested carbohydrates. As most intestinal bacteria are located in the colon, the patient with a colostomy will produce flatus formed in this way rather than by ingestion. The average length of time from eating flatus-producing foods to passing flatus from the colon is 6 h (Rideout 1987). Patients may choose to avoid these foods at certain times once this is understood.

Patients who experience a very loose stool with particular foods will need to take precautions, e.g. colostomists may need to use a drainable bag if eating foods known to cause diarrhoea.

Table 4.2 Possible effects of food on stoma function

Foods	Effect
Beans Beer Caffeinated beverages Chocolate Leafy green vegetables Raw fruits and vegetables Spicy foods Wholemeal food Cereals Alcohol Citrus fruits and juice Fried foods	May loosen stoma output
Apple sauce Bananas Boiled rice Cheese Tapioca White bread Potatoes Suet pudding Pasta Marshmallows Yoghurt	May thicken stoma output

Beer
Carbonated beverages
Dried beans and peas
Milk and milk products
Onions
Vegetables in the cabbage
  family (cabbage, broccoli,
  sprouts, sweetcorn)
	May cause flatus

Mushrooms Sweetcorn Potato skins Nuts Tomato skins Raw fruit skins/dried fruits Celery strings Oriental vegetables	Have been known to block ileostomies
Eggs Fish Onion family Pulses Root vegetables Spices	May produce odour

Food blockage

This is a potential problem for ileostomists, because the lumen of the small bowel is relatively narrow. Part-digested or undigested foods can become lodged in the lumen. The types of food that are likely to be the cause of a food blockage are high-fibre and stringy foods. Postoperatively, fibrous food is avoided, as at this time the oedema causes further narrowing. Eventually, fibrous foods can be introduced individually and their effects noted for the future.

Patients should be advised to chew all food thoroughly and to take plenty of fluids after swallowing food to ensure that food is 'washed through'.

Signs of food blockage

Partial obstruction. Cramping abdominal pain, offensive watery output, abdominal distension and swelling of the stoma may occur.

Patients who recognise the signs of partial food blockage can treat themselves by taking a warm bath, for relaxation and gentle massage, to try and relieve the pain and dislodge the obstruction. If they are not nauseated or vomiting, then oral fluids will help to dislodge the food. They are advised to contact their GP for advice.

Complete obstruction. In this case, nausea and vomiting, severe abdominal pain and distension, discolouration and swelling of the stoma occur with no output from the stoma. Complete obstruction requires hospitalisation for management.

SEXUAL DYSFUNCTION RELATED TO STOMA SURGERY

Loss or alteration in sexual function after surgery can be devastating for both the patient and the partner. Stoma formation often results from some degree of pelvic surgery. Pelvic surgery has the potential for disruption of the important (neurovascular) supply to the genitals. In males, this disruption may cause temporary or permanent impotence. In females, it may result in a lack of lubrication and expansion of the vagina. Extensive pelvic surgery such as proctectomy (removal of the rectum) and subsequent perineal scarring can make intercourse for females extremely painful. In removing the rectum during abdominoperineal excision, it may be necessary for the surgeon to remove part of the vaginal wall. Consequently, sexual intercourse may become painful or difficult and a change of position may be helpful.

It is important to establish the patient's understanding of the risks of surgery, and these will usually be explained by the surgeon and the stomatherapy nurse prior to consent. Eliciting the patient's sexual orientation, if possible, during the admission assessment is important, as there may be more far-reaching implications in some cases. For example, a homosexual male whose rectum is excised, may lose his sexual orifice and may also become impotent.

Where there is a high risk of impotence, it may be appropriate to discuss, pre-operatively, alternative methods of inducing erection, e.g. penile implants. This would be in conjunction with the stomatherapy nurse, the surgeon and a specialist in sexual dysfunction.

It should not be assumed that patients will accept the consequences of damaging pelvic surgery nor, indeed, that they will wish to pursue treatment for sexual dysfunction. This subject is often best dealt with after the patient and his partner have recovered from the situation and temporary loss of sexual function is ruled out. A satisfying sexual relationship can still be achieved without intercourse however, and patients and partners may even enjoy discovering their new sex life.

Sexuality and self-concept

Sexuality is both physical and emotional, is present throughout life and is constantly undergoing alteration. Many patients undergoing stoma surgery have anxiety as a result of sexual alterations. In a study on the quality of life for stoma patients, Wade (1989) found that some patients were too embarrassed to ask questions about sex and were not given an opportunity to do so. A caring and sympathetic nurse can make a difference to patients who feel that their sexuality is threatened.

Raising the issue of body image and self-concept gives patients permission to discuss their feelings, e.g.: 'The stoma is not difficult to deal with in practical terms but dealing with it in your mind may be more difficult.'

Patients do not always associate the loss if sexual desire with long-term illness or operation. They may solely blame the stoma. A partner who is reluctant to touch the new stoma patient intimately may be afraid of hurting him, but the patient may perceive this as a loss of attraction.

For a woman, the fact that an ileostomy may look phallic can affect her sense of femininity. For a man, bleeding from the stoma when caring for it may remind him of menstruation.

Stomal noises and bag rustling during intimate moments are valid worries; so too is the fear of the bag leaking. However, for Crohn's disease or ulcerative colitis sufferers, they may be less worrying than the fear of passing foulsmelling flatus, being incontinent during intercourse or having to rush away to the toilet. It is not infrequent for 'new' stoma patients to report an improvement in their sex lives due to feeling well for a change, and/or being able to relax during sex and not worry about these accidents. For females, tying a silky scarf around the waist to support and hide the stoma bag is an option.

All these issues need to be addressed as serious problems, but a sense of humour in the patient and her partner will help enormously during their adjustment. Coe & Kluka (1988) listed the concerns expressed by stoma patients and their partners related to social adjustment. These included concerns about being able to resume sexual activity; feeling alone; making changes in clothing styles; wondering how the stoma would affect daily activities; trying to sleep while wearing an appliance; having an unpleasant odour; passing wind; deciding whom to tell; and cleanliness.

The patient without a partner may find it difficult to enter into close relationships for fear of rejection. Patients need time to adjust to their stoma and the changes in their body before they can feel comfortable in sexual functioning. One particular young male ileostomist who has had several relationships in recent years reports that by the fifth or sixth date, he knows whether or not his new girlfriend will be able to accept the presence of the stoma. If he thinks she can, he will at this point show it to her.

SOCIAL SUPPORT

The support of another individual during times of crisis is instinctive in close relationships. However, the support network of each individual patient should be determined pre-operatively in order that strategies for postoperative care may be employed. Webster (1986) stated that patients with limited family and social support proved to be more vulnerable than others in terms of coping. For some, support may come in the form of a spouse who wishes to take on the care of the stoma. This situation is not infrequent and does not always receive positive outcomes, as dependence can be fostered which is impractical for stoma patients in some cases. However, Stewart (1985) stated that the very independent person is less likely to want to show her emotions. This scenario may not be conducive to problem-solving and discussing the issues related to the stoma that are most problematic to the patient.

Comprehensive care can only be given if the ability of willing 'significant others' to give care is assessed. Whether the care offered is emotional or practical, they too should receive information and support to assist them in providing this special care. Given the intimate and undesirable nature of stoma care, the strength of a relationship may be highlighted during rehabilitation. When one considers that a common initial reaction to the prospect of a stoma is the assumption that the partner will find them less attractive or unattractive, suggesting that the relationship may weaken or break, in fact, the opposite may be true.

Yaffe (1992) has suggested that, as with most traumatic life events, disease will find the weak spots or the strengths in people and their relationships. Nurses in gastroenterology may help in these situations by forming and maintaining a supportive relationship with the patient and carers.

THE ENTEROCUTANEOUS FISTULA

Definition

An enterocutaneous fistula is an abnormal communication between part of the gastrointestinal tract and the skin surface. Enterocutaneous fistulae can lead to rapid, life-threatening deterioration of the general condition of the patient with malnutrition, sepsis, electrolyte disturbances and dehydration (Rinsema 1994).

Enterocutaneous fistulae most commonly occur in patients with Crohn's disease, carcinoma, diverticular disease and those suffering damage to the bowel after radiation therapy.

According to Truscott (1992), 'Fistulae are the stomatherapist's nightmare and a fistula is most probably one of the worst and most upsetting complications a patient can endure.'

Whilst the latter part of the statement may be true, one of the most satisfying and rewarding situations for the gastroenterology nursing team is being equal to the demands of the all-encompassing, indiscriminate and untimely enterocutaneous fistula.

Most enterocutaneous fistulae occur after surgery, usually as a result of sepsis or a tenuous anastomosis. Rarely, the fistula forms spontaneously, usually in advanced carcinoma cases.

Historically, these fistulae have been associated with a high mortality rate and, until recent years, a poor prognosis (Devlin & Elcoat 1983). Conservative treatment was often inadequate in controlling the fistula and the sepsis, and in overcoming metabolic changes and preventing skin breakdown. Avoiding surgery in an already systematically compromised patient is preferable. These days, advances in diagnostic techniques and supportive care allow for a conservative approach with better success rates.

The method of management will be determined by the team and will depend on the characteristics and manifestation of the fistula.

Classifications of enterocutaneous fistulae relating to the type of appliance most suitable for management

Small-area fistula

This fistula involves a small area at skin level, possibly at the site of a previous incision, and it is possibly a spontaneous eruption due to abscess formation through a drain site. Effluent can be high or low in volume. It may be managed with a conventional stoma appliance and principles of stoma care.

Large-area fistula

This fistula involves a large surface area, e.g. a large dehisced laparotomy wound with further breakdown and possibly involvement of nearby drain sites. If the dehiscence extends down to the patient's pubic area, surface anatomy can be distorted on movement. A large stoma appliance and a number of accessory products may be indicated. Two smaller bags are often more flexible for the patient than one large one.

Low-output fistula

This fistula is usually from the lower gastrointestinal tract, e.g. a colocutaneous fistula in advanced carcinoma. It often functions as a colostomy or ileostomy and can therefore be managed with conventional stomatherapy appliances and principles of stoma care to ensure skin protection, comfort and security.

High-output fistula

This fistula is usually from the upper gastrointestinal tract and the effluent is therefore caustic due to proteolytic digestive enzymes. High output from a fistula is defined as a volume of more than 500 ml in 24 h. These fistulae usually pose management difficulties and intensive nursing time, as two people are required during 'dressing' changes. A secure appliance is essential as erythema has been reported within 2 h of skin contact and excoriation in 3–4 h. An appliance with a continuous drainage facility is indicated, along with a high durability skin protector.

Until the last two decades, high-output small bowel fistulae were considered to be uncontrollable with conservative measures. These days they are amenable to conservative medical treatment (e.g. TPN and octreotide to inhibit secretion) due to advances in supportive care, e.g. stomatherapy and nutrition nurse specialists, and the greater continuity afforded by the trend towards team and primary nursing (Pearson 1988).

Definitions of treatment measures (Rinsema 1994)

- *Primary conservative treatment* – measures intended to create optimal conditions for spontaneous closure of a gastrointestinal fistula or for delayed definitive surgery, e.g. skin and fistula care, nutrition, control of sepsis, diagnostic evaluation by contrast radiology or MRI.
- *Immediate operative treatment* – a definitive operation, performed within 1 week of the development of a fistula.
- *No treatment* – no conservative or operative treatment is started because of fistula- or patient-related factors.
- *Definitive operation* – operative procedure intended to eliminate the fistula, e.g. suture closure, resection with end-to-end anastomosis.
- *Delayed definitive operation* – definitive operation performed under stable conditions if conservative treatment did not result in spontaneous closure of the fistula.
- *Non-definitive operation* – operative procedures performed during conservative treatment not intended to close the fistula, but to create optimal conditions for spontaneous closure or delayed surgery, e.g. abscess drainage, creation of a defunctioning stoma, resection with exteriorization, partial or total bypass, operative placement of a catheter for enteral nutrition (jejunostomy), etc.

The primary conservative treatment of a high-output, large-area enterocutaneous fistula presents the most exacting challenge to the gastroenterology team. During this phase of treatment, the primary therapy is administered by the nursing team. Occasionally, reinfusion of the proximal effluent to the distal gut is advocated if the patient has suitable surface anatomy. Effluent collected from the proximal gut in a bag is infused via a catheter into the distal gut. The aim is to correct metabolic disturbances. Medical treatment to decrease the amount of effluent may also be advocated. Octreotide, for example, has been shown to decrease the output of fistulae when used as an adjuvant therapy during conservative management (Rinsema 1994).

Practical management (Fig. 4.7)

Each change in status of the fistula has far-reaching implications, e.g. an increase in output may undermine the security of a particular 'dressing' which will cause leakage onto the patient's skin. This may evoke feelings of loss of control for the patient, and the same feeling may be experienced by the nursing team who perhaps spent an hour or more securing the dressing. Persistent leakage will cause skin breakdown, malodour and pain, leading to low morale in the patient and the nurses. For the novice in fistula nursing, the first experience of a high-output fistula can be shocking.

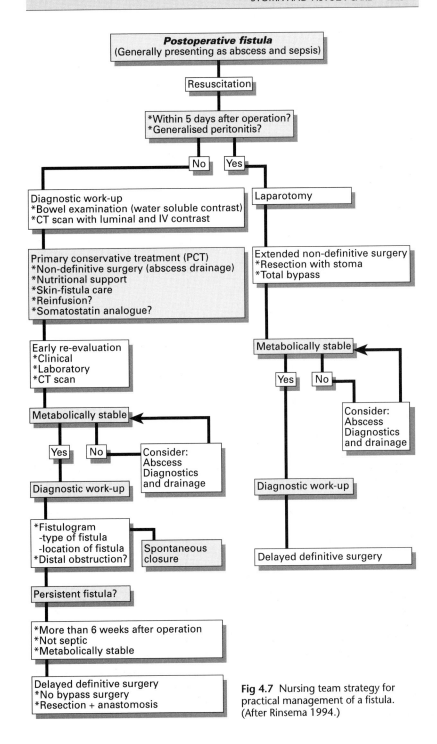

Fig 4.7 Nursing team strategy for practical management of a fistula. (After Rinsema 1994.)

Case history 4.3

Ann, a 26-year-old married woman with Crohn's disease, was admitted to the surgical ward for strictureplasty. Ann was forewarned that the operation would be lengthy and difficult, and that it may take her some weeks to recover from the effects of the long anaesthetic.

The operation was extremely problematic, the strictures were very dense and difficult to divide, and the intestine was perforating. As a result, the surgeon decided it would be unwise to close the abdomen, as Ann was very unstable clinically and the risk of sepsis would be too great.

After surgery, Ann's wound was discharging a high volume of small bowel effluent. The wound was approximately 17.5 cm wide and 20 cm long. The intestine was exposed. Ann's clinical status was addressed by the medical team and the following key aspects of nursing care were indentified:

- meticulous wound management to maintain skin integrity
- continuous drainage of effluent to prevent sepsis and further breakdown of abdominal wall
- maintenance of TPN to promote healing and general condition
- maintenance of Ann's self-esteem and morale
- teamwork.

The mortality rate for the patient with an enterocutaneous fistula is up to 20% (Lange et al 1989).

It was explained to Ann that she was seriously ill, and that her 'wound' would take many weeks to heal, if at all. Spontaneous closure of enterocutaneous fistulae occurs in up to 50% of cases (Lange et al 1989). Ann was allowed nothing by mouth. Total parenteral nutrition was commenced and the potential for line infection was recognised as high in this situation.

After careful assessment of the fistula site, it was clear that no single appliance was available to cover the wound adequately, therefore two Wound Managers (Convatec) were used. Other materials included filler paste, barrier wipes and Cohesive Seals (Salt & Son). Due to the nature and size of the wound, Ann was given sedation prior to commencing the dressing. A nurse sat with her to comfort and reassure her and to monitor her vital signs. Another nurse ensured that the effluent from the fistula did not come into contact with Ann's skin by using a suction catheter. It was recognised that Ann would be losing body heat with such a large area of her open abdomen exposed, and so she was wrapped up in blankets as much as possible.

A template of the wound was made by stretching a transparent abdominal dressing over Ann's abdomen and tracing the outline of the wound onto it.

Strips of backing paper were removed from the inside edges of two large Wound Managers side by side and stuck together. The template was carefully cut (see Fig. 4.8).

Indentations and wrinkles were filled with paste and Cohesive Seals were used to fill a deep crease at the bottom of the wound in her pubic area. The paste was dried using piped oxygen to speed up the setting process. When the paste was dry, two nurses positioned the 'dressing' accurately, whilst another maintained the continuous suction at this crucial moment.

After positioning and smoothing down, paste was added using a syringe to

---

Case history 4.3 *(cont'd)*

improve the skin/Wound Manager contact in areas where Ann's distorted abdomen was lifting it slightly.

As the output was in excess of 3 L, a low-pressure pump suction was advocated. One of these was laid on either side of the wound and exited the Wound Managers via the drainage ports; they were attached to two suction bottles, one on either side of Ann's bed. The flatus filters on the windows of the Wound Managers were covered with waterproof tape to help prevent odour caused by seepage. Warm sterile saline and iodine solution was trickled over the wound through the window of the Wound Manager on a daily basis to remove static debris from the wound edges (see Fig. 4.9).

On average, the dressing remained intact for 3 days before renewal was necessary. It took two nurses approximately $1\frac{1}{2}$ hours from beginning to end. After a few weeks, Ann was able to participate, holding the suction catheter in her wound.

There was a slight odour about Ann which mostly came from the suction bottles, and she was understandably low in spirits; she felt unattractive, she missed her family and she could not see an end to the situation.

Ann eventually left the ward after 9 months, during which time the fistula dressing was modified according to the size, shape and output. Familiarity with the products is essential as they can be awkward to apply and costly to waste.

Procedures such as the one above are more efficiently carried out with two nurses in order to maintain continuous suction, thus keeping the effluent under control. When appropriate, a Foley catheter may be used to stem the flow of effluent from a fistula by careful insertion and inflating the balloon with water.

One of the most difficult aspects of caring for a patient with a complicated fistula is the maintenance of patient, relatives and staff morale. There is no doubt that it is very demoralising for all when the dressing fails. Progress is often slow as the drainage is unremitting. Advanced nursing skills must be employed to provide the necessary positive reassurance to keep the patient hopeful.

Complicated fistulae are more efficiently dressed by those who are familiar with them and this is the tendency. Therefore, it can be very emotionally draining on individual nurses and this is why a supportive team is essential.

After the diagnosis of the fistula, and conservative treatment has been 'prescribed' (see Fig. 4.7), a nursing team strategy for practical management should be employed, taking into consideration the immediate and long-term needs of the patient (see Case history 4.3). Sharing past experience of this type of fistula could be construtive, especially for novices.

Initial assessment of fistula

Nature of fistula effluent

The more proximal the fistula, the more damaging is its effect on the patient's skin and abdominal wall. Effluent containing activated gastric, biliary or pan-

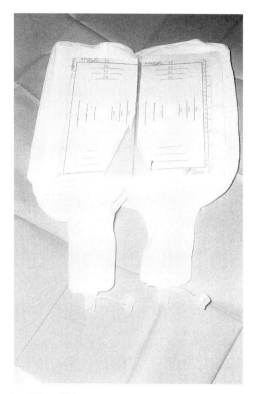

Fig 4.8 Joining two Wound Managers.

creatic juice may cause rapid digestion of skin, pain, infection and evasion of deeper layers.

Irving & Beadle (1982) classifies the skin condition of fistulae into the following categories:

- *one* – the fistula is a single orifice passing through an intact abdominal wall or otherwise healed scar, surrounded by flat skin in a reasonably good condition
- *two* – the fistula has a single or multiple orifices passing through the abdominal wall close to bony prominences, surgical scars, other stomas or the umbilicus
- *three* – the fistula has an orifice situated in a small dehiscence of the abdominal wound
- *four* – the fistula has an orifice situated in a large dehiscence of the abdominal wall or at the bottom of a gaping wound

A 'map' of the abdominal surface drawn on the nursing care plan is helpful, with approximate or actual measurements. Broken or reddened areas of

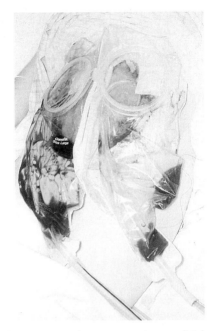

Fig 4.9 Use of Wound Manager on a large enterocutaneous fistula.

skin should also be noted as potential sites of pain or lacking in adherent properties.

Where possible, viewing the abdomen with the patient lying and sitting may reveal a distorted skin surface which may be a complicating factor.

Finding a suitable 'dressing technique'

A wide range of materials is available in hospitals under 'stoma care products'. Large 'postoperative' stoma bags, high-output drainage bags, wound managers, skin protective sheets, filler pastes, etc. are all possibilities (see Fig. 4.4).

Finding the most suitable appliance will depend on the volume and type of effluent, and the size and shape of the fistula.

A combination of dressings may be appropriate. For instance, packing and covering some areas 'upstream' of the discharge in a large wound may make it easier to contain the high-output area in a smaller drainage bag. In this way, some areas of the fistula wound may be offered greater protection from the caustic effluent. The patient's comfort and degree of mobility are, of course, important considerations; smaller appliances are more flexible.

There is no standard method of applying drainage bags to fistulae as each one is unique. Ingenuity and creativity are required by the nursing team, and experience is definitely a bonus (see Case history 4.3).

REFERENCES

Alterescu V 1985 Stoma lacerations. Journal of Enterostomal Therapy 12:217
Brooke B N 1952 The management of an ileostomy including its complications. *Lancet* 2:102
Corney R 1991 Developing communications and counselling skills in medicine. Tavistock/Routledge, London, ch 1
Coe M, Kluka S 1988 Concerns of clients and spouses regarding ostomy surgery for cancer. Journal of Enterostomal Therapy 15:232
Cuschieri A, Giles G R, Moosa A R 1988 The colon, rectum and anal canal. Essential Surgical Practice 74, 1203, Wright, London.
Devlin H B 1982 Stomatherapy review, part 3. Coloproctology 5:298–306
Devlin H B, Elcoat C E 1983 Alimentary tract fistula: stomatherapy techniques of management. World Journal of Surgery 7
Goligher J 1984 Surgery of the anus, rectum and colon, 5th edn. Baillière Tindall, London, ch 18, p 568
Irving M, Beadle C H 1982 External intestinal fistulae: nursing care & surgical procedures. Clinics in Gastroenterology 11:327–336
Kelly M P 1992 Colitis. Tavistock/Routledge, London, ch 4, p 54
Lange M P, Thebo L M, Tiede S M, McCarthy B, Dahn M, Jacobs L A 1989 Management of multiple enterocutaneous fistulae. Heart and Lung 18(4):386–391
Pearson A 1988 Primary nursing. Croom Helm, London
Rideout B 1987 The patient with an ileostomy: nursing management and education. Nursing Clinics of North America 22:253
Rinsema W 1994 Gastrointestinal fistulae: management & results of treatment. Datawyse, Maastricht
Roy C 1984 Introduction to nursing: an adaptation model. Prentice Hall, London
Stewart W 1985 Counselling in rehabilitation. Croom Helm, London, ch 10
Truscott J 1992 Management profile: fistulae. WCET Journal 12(2):9
Wade B 1989 A stoma is for life. Scutari Press Inc, London
Webster M 1986 Patients' coping strategies. Nursing Times, October 22
Yaffe A 1992 Family members as caregivers – their influence on stoma patients' self care. WCET Journal 12:25–27

USEFUL TELEPHONE NUMBERS

British Colostomy Association: 01734 391537
The Ileostomy and Internal Pouch Support Group: 01623 28099
Urostomy Association: 01245 224924
National Association for Colitis and Crohn's Disease: 01727 844296

Gastrointestinal bleeding

Margaret Butler

This chapter will consider the management of patients with acute and chronic gastrointestinal (GI) haemorrhage, the causes of haemorrhage, the treatment options and the implications for patients' future lives.

UPPER GASTROINTESTINAL BLEEDING

Acute upper gastrointestinal bleeding is one of the most common medical emergencies, accounting for over 28 000 admissions to hospitals in the UK each year (Morris 1992). A district general hospital, for example, serving a population of 250 000 would expect to admit approximately four patients per week with haematemesis or melaena.

The 1970s saw the introduction of fibre-optic endoscopy, which improved diagnostic accuracy but did not alter the mortality from GI bleeding. In fact, the overall mortality has remained almost constant over the last 50 years at around 10% (Allan & Dykes 1976, Cutler & Mendeloff 1981). The admission of patients to designated bleeding units decreases the mortality to 4–6%, not least because of the specialist nursing care such patients receive. It is possible that one of the main reasons for this continued high mortality is the progressively increasing age of the population (Hunt et al 1979, Morris 1992).

The main causes of upper GI bleeding in patients in the UK are listed in Box 5.1 and some are shown in Figure 5.1.

It is important to note that the proportion of cases with oesophageal variceal bleeding is greater in countries where alcohol consumption is higher and where hepatitis B virus infection is common. Upper GI bleeding has also become increasingly associated with the taking of non-steroidal anti-inflammatory drugs (NSAIDs), for arthritis or painful locomotor disorders. In one study of patients bleeding from peptic ulceration, almost 35% had taken NSAIDs in the week prior to presentation, with 84% of them being over 60 years of age (Holman et al 1990).

Box 5.1 Causes of upper gasrointestinal bleeding (after Morris 1992)

Common
Duodenal and gastric ulceration
Oesophagitis
Gastritis
Duodenitis
Varices
Mallory–Weiss tear

Less common
Carcinomas
Bleeding diathesis
Leiomyomas
Aortic aneurysm fistula

Rare (less than 1%)
Dieulafoy lesion
Angiomas
Hereditary haemorrahagic telangiectasia
Pseudoxanthoma elasticum
Ehlers–Danlos syndrome
Haemobilia
Pancreatic bleeding
Foreign body

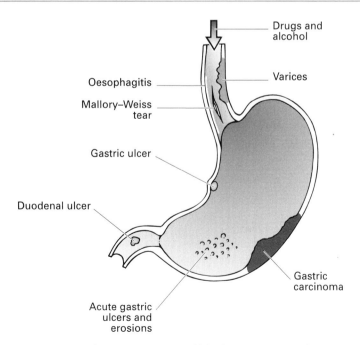

Fig 5.1 Some causes of upper gastrointestinal bleeding in patients in the UK.

Causes of upper GI bleeding

Peptic ulceration is the most common cause of upper GI bleeding, accounting for 55% of all cases.

Peptic ulcers are defects in the gastrointestinal mucosae which occur as a result of pepsin and acid activity. The extent of this defect can be right through the muscularis mucosae. Ulcers can be grouped into three categories, depending on their cause:

1. *Helicobacter pylori* associated ulcers
2. ulcers caused by NSAIDs, such as aspirin
3. stress ulcers.

There are other categories, but they are rare and beyond the scope of this text.

H. Pylori

H. Pylori is a bacterium found mainly in the antrum of the stomach; it is thought to be one of the most common infections worldwide. The differences in the prevalence of *H. pylori* infection in differing populations is dramatic. The developing world has a much higher incidence than the Western world (Graham 1991). In the Western world, the incidence is much higher in blacks than in whites, and it is also higher in lower socio-economic groups than in higher ones. There is a trend towards increasing prevalence with age in developing countries. For example, in the USA whites show a prevalence of 10–20% below 30 years of age; this increases steadily at the rate of about 1% per year, to greater than 50% by age 60 (Graham et al 1991).

The association between *H. pylori* and peptic ulcer disease is now widely accepted, but the mechanism of the pathology remains unclear (Sleisenger & Fordtran 1993).

Treatment of *H. pylori* is effective using drug co-therapy. The recommendations for these therapies are reviewed frequently; readers are advised to consult their local gastroenterology department for current policies. The following example (in practice at the time of going to press) of such a therapy taken for 1 week achieves up to 93% eradication (Oxford Radcliffe Trust, unpublished work, 1996):

omeprazole	20 mg bd
clarithromycin	250 mg bd
metronidazole	400 mg bd

Non-steroidal anti-inflammatory drugs

NSAIDs are thought to be ulcerogenic due to the reduction in mucosal prostaglandin production. Prostaglandins inhibit acid secretion as well as enhancing mucosal defence. Treatment and prevention of such ulcers can be successful using a co-therapy of prostaglandin analogue (e.g. misoprostol) with an H_2 blocker (e.g. ranitidine) (Lanza et al 1989).

Stress ulcers

Many people and their doctors are convinced that peptic ulcer disease is exacerbated by stressful life events. The importance of psychodynamic factors in the development of peptic ulcer, however, remains a controversy. The study of such an influence has been extensive, but is hampered by difficulties in defining stress, ulcer disease sampling and in finding 'unstressed' controls (Tennant 1988).

Anecdotal evidence, however, suggests there is a link; for example, following the Blitz 1941, there was a reported increase in the number of perforated peptic ulcers (Spicer et al 1944). In another study, 25% of prisoners of war developed duodenal ulcers during follow-up, compared with 11% of the control group, who had not been captured. These examples suggest a causal link with stress. Proof, as mentioned before, is difficult to establish.

Other causes

Associated factors thought to exacerbate peptic ulceration include cigarette smoking, high concentrations of alcohol intake and certain ulcerogenic foodstuffs, such as refined rice (Malhotra 1978).

Most upper GI bleeds are a result of chronic gastric or duodenal ulcers (DUs). Although duodenal ulcers are four times more common than gastric ulcers, the incidence of GI bleeding from DU is not quadrupled. Indeed, DUs account for 35% of upper GI bleeds, manifested by haematemesis or malaena and GUs for 20% of upper GI bleeds (Travis et al 1993).

Other causes are far less common: Mallory–Weiss tear accounts for 6% of upper GI bleeds. This is a mucosal tear at the oesophagogastric junction due to forceful vomiting, often following excess alcohol.

Duodenitis and gastritis each account for less than 5% of the incidence of upper GI bleeding. Oesophageal varices, too, make up only 5% of all upper GI bleeding cases. Any other causes each contribute less than 1% to the whole picture.

NURSING MANAGEMENT OF A PATIENT WITH UPPER GI BLEEDING

It is important to remember that most GI bleeds stop spontaneously. Of peptic ulcers, about 20% will rebleed in hospital and many of these will require surgical intervention. The nursing management of these patients is detailed below. The emphasis is on nursing as part of the core team in resuscitating and maintaining the patient prior to endoscopy and/or surgery.

Assessment

It is important to assess the patient for:

- signs of hypovolaemia or shock
- clues to the cause of the haemorrhage (see Table 5.1).

The initial management depends on the clinical state of the patient.

The main initial priority should be to resuscitate the patient and preserve oxygenation of vital organs. It is important to remember that most patients who present with GI bleeding are, at least initially, conscious and aware of their surroundings and that they are haemorrhaging. It is a terrifying experience for them and their families, and so constant reassurance and explanations are vital.

Table 5.1 Physical signs as clues to the causes of upper GI bleeding (after Morris 1992

Clinical features	Possible GI abnormality
Signs of portal hypertension	Varices
Telangiectasia (lips, tongue)	Gastroduodenal telangiectasia
Signs of bleeding diathesis	Mucosal bleeding or varices
Arthritis	Peptic ulceration or gastritis
Weight loss	Carcinoma, gastric ulcer
Epigastric mass	Carcinoma
Abnormal skin (elasticity/scarring)	Pseudoxanthoma elasticum/ Ehlers–Danlos syndrome

The value of psychosocial assessment is vital at this stage, to gain insight into the most effective reassurance measures and to facilitate fuller understanding of the patient and their family. The significance of continuity of care, provided within an individualised approach, cannot be overemphasised.

Resuscitation

Note blood pressure and pulse rate, as well as postural drop on sitting up (>15 mm Hg drop indicates a high-risk patient) and signs of sympathetic overactivity, including sweating and pallor. Thirst is also a major symptom in a hypovolaemic patient. If there is uncertainty about hypovolaemia, the medical staff will normally consider central venous pressure (CVP) monitoring or the insertion of a Swann–Ganz catheter, to optimise fluid management and monitor changes in systemic vascular resistance. Hypovolaemia must be treated promptly. If the patient is hypovolaemic, he/she will have:

- tachycardia and/or other signs of sympathetic overactivity
- low blood pressure – this is a late sign, especially in the young, when it may be too late to be able to resuscitate.

It is important that large-bore venous access is obtained and consideration is given as to whether central venous pressure monitoring is required. CVP monitoring is usually considered for patients when fluctuations in fluid volume may compromise one or more systems, such as:

- those requiring large volumes of blood
- patients with cardiac problems
- patients with renal problems
- patients with respiratory problems
- the elderly.

Even if these patients are not in shock, they tolerate transfusion less well and are at risk of developing heart failure from fluid overload.

The patient should be nursed as flat as can be tolerated and should have oxygen administered. The following blood tests will be required:

- FBC
- platelet count
- prothrombin time
- liver function tests
- urea and electolytes
- blood for cross-matching.

Intravenous fluid replacement will be needed, specifically blood, as soon as it is available (to maintain oxygen-carrying capacity) to raise the CVP to normal (0 to +10). While awaiting cross-matched blood, either synthetic plasma expander or crystalloids may be used. If vital signs do not improve despite adequate blood replacement, or if the patient continues to bleed with large fresh haematemesis, urgent surgical assessment is needed.

At this point, the patient and her family have to consider the added risk of surgery. Continuous reassurance, explanation and, when possible, opportunities to discuss decisions to be made with the medical and nursing staff will contribute to their comfort. Indications for surgery are as follows:

- >4 units transfused (age > 60 years)
- >8 units transfused (age < 60 years)
- continued bleeding
- rebleed in hospital.

Once resuscitated, if surgery is not required, the patient usually undergoes endoscopy within hours to identify the source of the blood loss. Apart from hypovolaemia, patients may require blood transfusions for:

- observed loss of large amounts of blood
- initial haemoglobin < 10 g/dl.

All patients bleeding from the upper GI tract should have nil orally until they have a diagnostic endoscopy. Endoscopy can usually be performed on the next available elective list, particularly where criteria are fulfilled for emergency endoscopy in specialised units, e.g. continued bleeding; rebleeding in hospital; in patients with coexistent hepatic disease; and where a surgical decision depends on the outcome of endoscopy. Figure 5.2 illustrates a summary of suggested management for acute upper GI bleeds.

If no lesion is seen at endoscopy and the bleeding is not considered serious, the patient is likely to be discharged. Many such patients are young and the bleed has been asscociated with an alcoholic binge. It is important that their awareness of alcohol-related illness is assessed and appropriate information given prior to discharge. Whilst patients cannot be made to change their lifestyles, nurses can help to ensure that they have enough information and support to facilitate such a change should they wish.

Older patients with definite but small haematemesis and negative endoscopy may be discharged but kept under review in the outpatient clinic.

An increased risk of mortality has been associated with:

- age over 60 years
- continued or recurrent bleeding

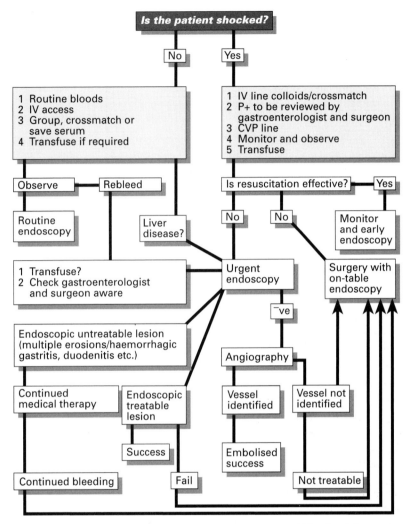

Fig 5.2 Suggested management of acute upper gastrointestinal bleeding (after Morrris 1992).

- presence of other serious concomitant disease
- ulcer pain persisting after admission
- NSAID use
- gastric rather than duodenal ulceration
- chronic rather than acute ulceration.

It is important to be aware of these factors, especially when explaining the importance of medication to patients and the effect on their lifestyle.

There are two main endoscopic therapies of established value:

- *Thermal techniques* – designed to produce local heat at the point of bleeding to coagulate proteins and cause their contraction. This shrinkage of tissue to narrow the vascular lumen is the major haemostatic mechanism, with secondary thrombosis within the vessel.
- *Injection therapy*
  — Adrenaline produces its haemostatic effect mainly by vasoconstriction with added platelet aggregation
  — sclerosants produce their effects by direct vascular thrombosis with secondary surrounding fibrosis.

Snyman et al (1992) pointed out that:

- about 70–80% of peptic ulcers spontaneously stop bleeding and do not rebleed
- only 1–2% of patients will require immediate surgery to control exsanguination
- about 25% of patients will require urgent surgery for recurrent or continued bleeding, usually within 72 hours of admission.

Pharmacological therapy (such as H_2 receptor antagonists), while playing no role in stopping bleeding, has an important place in preventing stress ulcers in critically ill patients. Maintenance therapy reduces the incidence and symptoms of recurrent ulceration, but does not necessarily prevent late rebleeding (Snyman et al 1992).

Some of the surgical options for treating upper GI bleeds are listed below:

- The main operation is *undersewing the bleeding vessel* for duodenal ulcers. This stops the bleeding. Other surgical techniques are designed to aid ulcer healing and prevent recurrence.
- *Truncal vagotomy and pyloroplasty* – this is still one of the operations of choice in the UK for bleeding (Stringer & Cameron 1988).
- *Truncal vagotomy and adtrectomy and Billroth I reconstruction* (see Figure 5.3).
- *Billroth II gastrectomy* – this may be required to control bleeding especially after rebleeding following a more conservative operation. (NB – suture line leakage and duodenal stump complications are major sources of morbidity and mortality, limiting the indications for this type of operation.)
- *Conventional surgery* – gastrectomy, usually of Billroth II type. It is associated with little risk of rebleeding and low risk of ulcer recurrence (4%), but has a relatively high mortality of 16% (Ovaska & Havia 1988). This will be increased in high-risk groups such as the elderly.

The widespread use of endoscopy and improved pharmacological prevention and treatment therapies have reduced the need for some surgical procedures.

Oesophageal varices

Increased portal vascular resistance leads to a gradual reduction in the flow of portal blood to the liver and simultaneously to the development of collateral vessels, allowing portal blood to bypass the liver and enter the systemic circulation directly. Collateral vessel formation occurs mainly in the GI tract, espe-

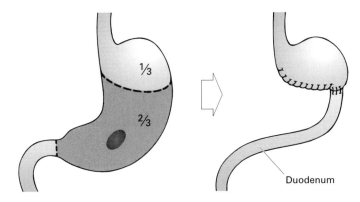

A Billroth I gastrectomy

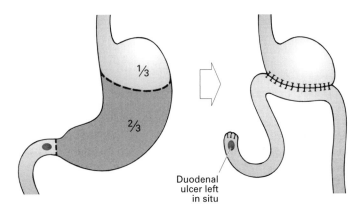

B Polya type gastrectomy

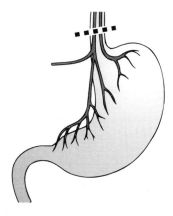

C Trunkal vagotomy

Fig 5.3 A: Billroth I gastrectomy. B: Polya-type gastrectomy. C: Trunkal vagotomy (after Burkitt et al 1990).

cially the oesophagus, stomach and rectum. The oesaphageal collaterals are known as oesophageal varices.

Bleeding from oesophageal varices may be rapid and exsanguinating, requiring urgent treatment for its control and resuscitation of the patient. It is also worth noting that the patient's general condition may already be poor because of previous haemorrhage and impairment of renal and hepatic function.

A first bleed carries a mortality of between 20 and 40%, and even once bleeding is controlled, the patient stands a more than 70% chance of a second major haemorrhage within a year.

There are a number of treatment options concentrating on controlling an acute bleeding episode and preventing rebleeding in the future. Bleeding from varices is a terrifying experience for patients and their families and, once again, constant reassurance and explanations are crucial to their psychological support.

Resuscitation

This should be commenced immediately. The patient will need blood, while avoiding overtransfusion by monitoring the CVP. Fresh frozen plasma and platelets are also generally required to correct deficiencies in coagulation caused by hepatic decompensation and the need to give donated blood (which lacks clotting factors). All patients should be nursed in a high dependency or specialist unit for GI haemorrhage.

Endoscopy

This is essential to confirm that (1) varices are present; (2) they are the source of the bleeding. The varices appear as bluish protrusions into the oesophageal lumen. They tend to be most visible at, or above the gastro-oesophageal junction.

Once varices are confirmed, the patient should ideally be transferred to a specialist centre when the bleeding has been controlled and resuscitation completed. Further measures may be required to prevent recurrence. The possibility of a transfer further heightens the anxiety of the patient and their family.

Shields (1992) suggested that endoscopy on admission be mandatory and, if active bleeding is confirmed, treatment is begun immediately with injection of the varices with sclerosant. Urgent treatment with sclerotherapy avoids the use of vasoactive drugs (and their side-effects) and balloon tamponade, which are markedly inferior.

Endoscopic injection sclerotherapy is currently the most popular method of controlling acute variceal haemorrhage. Up to 90% of acute bleeds can be controlled by endoscopic sclerotherapy (Shields 1992).

There are a number of variations in endoscopic sclerotherapy, such as intravariceal or paravariceal injection, type of sclerosant, volumes of sclerosant or sedation. Complications can include ulceration at the site of injection (more common after paravariceal than after intravariceal injection), oesophageal stricture (easily dilated) and, rarely, perforation of the oesophagus. The patient may be slightly pyrexial after the procedure and complain of dull, retrosternal pain and discomfort for 24 h. This is due to oesophageal reaction to the sclerosant.

Rebleeding. In about 10–15% of patients, rebleeding may occur within hours or days of initial treatment and may require blood transfusion. In such cases further endoscopy will be necessary.

Endoscopic band ligation offers the option of a treatment that can be applied during the mandatory diagnostic gastrointestinal endoscopy performed on anyone presenting with a variceal bleed. This may be more effective than sclerotherapy in controlling bleeding from large varices.

Causes of rebleeding are:

- recurrent bleeding from oesophageal varices
- bleeding from gastric varices
- bleeding from oesophageal ulcer secondary to injection
- bleeding from oesophagitis, gastric erosion or portal hypertensive gastropathy.

If the previously injected varices are the bleeding source, an octreotide infusion may be needed. If the bleeding is from oesophageal varices after octreotide treatment, repeat endoscopic sclerotherapy is indicated. If the bleeding remains uncontrolled, surgery is considered urgent if the patient's condition and liver function permit.

Vasoactive drugs

Vasopressin
- Powerful systemic and splanchnic vasoconstrictor
- Reduces portal pressure and flow
- Usually given as a continuous intravenous infusion
- Rarely used in most centres.

Generalised vasoconstriction may cause problems such as coronary, cerebral and mesenteric vasoconstriction, which may lead to infarction of the related tissues and organs. If problems occur, treatment with vasopressin will have to be stopped. Bleeding is only controlled in about 50–60% of episodes (Shields, 1992). To maximise benefits of vasopressin and to reduce complications it is sometimes combined with nitroglycerin.

Octreotide. This seems to act by reducing the flow and pressure in the collateral circulation (e.g. oesophageal varices), rather than reducing portal pressure directly. It works as well as vasopressin but has substantially fewer side-effects.

Balloon tamponade

This is only used when it has not been possible to control bleeding by sclerotherapy. It allows time for resuscitation and treatment planning, and it can be effective in stopping bleeding in 70–80% of patients. Use of an oesophageal balloon should be discontinued after 12–24 h only, to avoid necrosis of the oesophagus. This type of balloon is rarely used now (a gastric balloon alone is sufficient in >90%). When the tube is removed, there is a high rate of recurrence of bleeding. If bleeding continues during tamponade, it indicates that there is bleeding from other sites such as fundal varices, gastric ulcer or possibly coagulation problems.

Patients are at risk of developing serious complications such as oesophageal necrosis and rupture and aspiration pneumonia. Shields (1992) and Leicester (1990) put the estimate at 10%.

A number of different tubes are available, one of the most popular being the Minnesota modification of the Sengstaken–Blakemore tube. This has four channels; the longest one is used for aspirating the stomach, the second longest for inflating the gastric balloon, the third longest for inflating the sausage-shaped oesophageal balloon and the shortest for aspirating blood and swallowed saliva (pharyngeal) (see Fig. 5.4). A pair of scissors kept beside the patient enables the tube to be cut and quickly removed should the oesophageal balloon migrate into the hypopharynx or if respiratory distress develops. The patient should always be effectively sedated and may sometimes need ventilation to protect the airway.

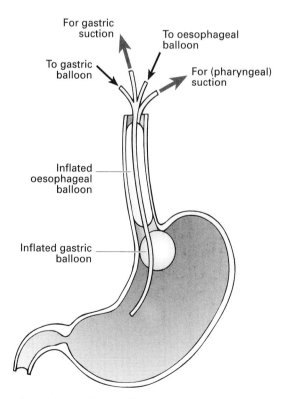

Fig 5.4 Sengstaken–Blakemore tube in situ.

Whilst the tube is in situ, communication will be difficult for the patient, and aids for non-verbal communication may be useful, such as a picture board or wipe board and pen. Skin traction on the tube and pressure in the balloon should be recorded every 4 h and maintained at about 20–30 mmHg.

A balloon tamponade is very distressing for patients and their families. Continuity of care is vital in these situations, in order to establish a relationship with the patient and family. This will help create trust and reassurance, to enable them to cope with the situation and to give them a key person to whom they may turn for support.

Bleeding gastric varices

These can be temporarily controlled by balloon tamponade. The gastric balloon will need to be well inflated with moderate traction, as gastric varices are normally high in the fundus. Sclerotherapy can be used but is often ineffective. Surgery will be required in many cases. The mortality is high (~50%).

Surgery

The following are surgical options in the treatment of oesophageal varices, although the outcomes of emergency surgical procedures in a jaundiced patient with hypoalbuminaemia, ascites and encephalopathy is extremely poor.

Oesophageal transection. This involves stapling the transection of the oesophagus in an attempt to obliterate the varices. The oesophagus is simultaneously transected and re-anastomosed. This procedure avoids the increased risk of encephalopathy associated with shunt operations.

Portal systemic shunt. This aims to reduce portal pressure and so control the haemorrhage and prevent recurrent bleeding. A major anastomosis between splanchic and systemic veins is required. Shunt operations usually stop the haemorrhage and prevent recurrence but they increase the risk of hepatoportal encephalopathy and postoperative liver failure. This is because the liver is bypassed and there is no detoxification of the blood.

They are generally divided into two types:

1. total portasystemic shunts, e.g. end-to-side portacaval shunt, M-graft portacaval shunt, mesocaval shunt and central splenorenal shunts; the entire splanchic bed is decompressed (Fig. 5.5)
2. selective shunts – the gastro-oesophageal varices are provided with a selective decompressive pathway, while portal hypertension is maintained in the rest of the splanchic circulation.

It is hoped in these operations that the venous blood flow to the liver is preserved, and with hepatic perfusion unimpaired, liver function does not deteriorate postoperatively because of the shunt.

There is increasing consideration being given to referring some of these patients for assessment for liver transplantation. This creates a whole new set of accompanying psychological needs for patients and their family which are beyond the scope of this text.

The development of transjugular intrahepatic portasystemic stent shunts

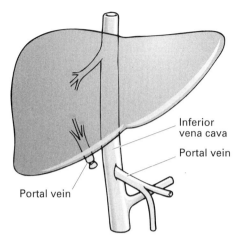

Fig 5.5 End-to-side portacaval shunt (after Taylor et al 1984).

(TIPSS) has created an additional option for the management of variceal bleeds.

Shunts (via TIPSS) are created within the liver by the passage of a needle or stylet from an hepatic vein into the portal vein branch using a transjugular approach via the superior vena cava. After the connection has been made, the tract is dilated by balloon angioplasty and a metallic stent is inserted to maintain patency. TIPSS provides a means of creating an intrahepatic shunt while avoiding surgery. It can be used to stop active bleeding as well as to prevent recurrent variceal bleeding. It can also be undertaken in severely ill patients who are unlikely to be fit for surgery.

Preventing complications
• Lactulose may be given to minimise or prevent hepatoportal encephalopathy. Lactulose increases acidity of stools, preventing formation of nitrogenous compounds whilst neomycin may also be given to reduce the presence of bacteria, although there is no proven additional benefit.
• Gastric erosion or peptic ulceration may be prevented by the administration of H_2 antagonist or proton pump inhibitor drugs.
• Renal failure due to hypotension after haemorrhage must be prevented. Resuscitation should be with blood or salt-poor albumin as breakdown of aldosterone is affected by liver failure and leads to intravascular retention of water. Fluids may be restricted if plasma concentration of Na^+ <130 mmol/L.
  — Paracentesis will be accompanied by infusion of salt-poor albumin in the presence of ascites:
  — no diuretics should be given if the patient is hypovolaemic or in shock.
  — 24-h urine measurement.
  — maintain CVP between +4 and +8 cmH_2O.

- Coagulation should be maintained with platelets and fresh frozen plasma if necessary.
- Infections should be identified and treated immediately.

Little prophylactic treatment can be offered to varices patients. However, propranolol is often prescribed in a dose that reduces the resting pulse rate by 25% as it decreases the risk of bleeding by reducing portal pressure. However, it has little effect on mortality and can be difficult for patients to tolerate due to side effects.

LOWER GASTROINTESTINAL BLEEDING

Massive bleeding from the lower GI tract is uncommon. The most common causes of lower gastrointestinal bleeding are minor anorectal conditions such as anal fissure or haemorrhoids. These conditions rarely cause major acute blood loss, although they should always be excluded as a source of bleeding. Colorectal polyps, colorectal carcinoma and ulcerative colitis are other common causes of lower GI bleeding. Extensive blood loss from an upper GI lesion can rarely present as rectal bleeding.

Drug therapy may also cause bleeding (usually occult) e.g. NSAIDs may cause a small bowel enteropathy and poorly controlled anticoagulant therapy may precipitate significant bleeding from malignancies and minor mucosal lesions (see Fig 5.6).

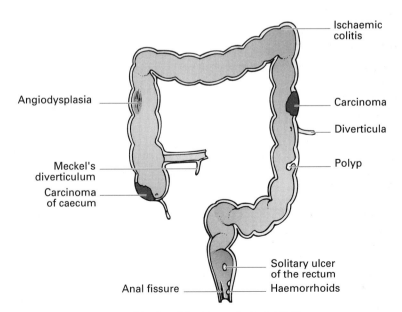

Fig 5.6 Causes of lower GI bleeding (after Kumar & Clark 1989).

Presentation
- Bright red rectal bleeding (a distal lesion)
- Dark red rectal bleeding (which may be mixed with mucus if an inflammatory or neoplastic lesion).

Other possible causes
- History of abdominal pain and altered bowel habit may indicate a malignancy.
- Diarrhoea may indicate inflammation (NB – bloody diarrhoea is entirely distinct from rectal bleeding with a change in bowel habit).
- Recent overseas travel, especially to areas where amoebic or schistosomal infections are common, should be noted as there may be an infection.
- Diverticular disease.
- Radiotherapy, even if a number of years ago, can cause radiation colitis.
- Elderly patients with cardiovascular disease may have ischaemic colitis or angiodysplasia (see Box 5.2).
- Ischaemic colitis is also a possible cause after aortic aneurysm surgery or mesenteric infarction.
- No cause identified.

Whilst obtaining a thorough history from patients is important in ensuring rapid appropriate diagnosis and treatment for the medical staff, a thorough nursing assessment ensures prompt and appropriate care for already anxious patients and relatives.

Box 5.2 Causes of lower gastrointestinal bleeding

Anorectal conditions
Haemorrhoids
Anal fissure
Solitary benign rectal ulcer

Children
Meckel's diverticulum
Juvenile polyps
Inflammatory bowel disease

Adults
Inflammatory bowel disease
Adenomatous polyps
Carcinoma
Arteriovenous malformation

Elderly
Carcinoma
Diverticular disease
Angiodysplasia
Adenomatous polyps
Ischaemic colitis
Inflammatory bowel disease

Resuscitation

Resuscitation may be vital in patients presenting with acute lower GI bleeds. Once completed, certain investigations will be considered.

Investigations

- Rectal examination, digital examination to palpate rectal lesions, e.g. carcinoma
- Proctoscopy, by using disposable proctoscope to examine the rectum, e.g. for haemorrhoids
- Sigmoidoscopy – flexible or rigid endoscopy to examine the sigmoid colon, e.g. for inflammatory bowel disease
- Barium enema – will show any mucosal lesion
- Colonoscopy – enables diagnosis and removal of any polyps in one procedure; this is preferable to a barium enema for visible rectal bleeding
- Angiography – shows vascular abnormality, e.g. angiodysplasia (rarely necessary)
- Under exceptional circumstances, laparotomy with intraoperative colonoscopy is carried out to identify and treat the problem in one procedure.

Severe bleeding stops spontaneously in 80% of cases after adequate blood replacement (Travis et al 1993). It is important, however, that the cause is treated. If bleeding is continuous or recurs, the site needs to be identified and surgery is usually considered.

Surgery

Options for surgery are

- laparotomy
- segmental resection if the site is identified
- 'blind' (R) hemicolectomy if the site cannot be identified and the patient is elderly (in such patients the cause may well be angiodysplasia in the proximal colon).

Surgery is, however, avoided where possible.

Haemorrhoids may be treated with rubber band ligation, injection, or infrared coagulation. Acute ulcerative colitis and Crohn's disease are dealt with in Chapter 4. Bleeding from radiation colitis may be more difficult to control, and requires resection in severe cases. It may respond to steroid enemas. Ischaemic colitis is usually self-limiting, although it may lead to stricture formation.

Infective colitis is best treated with appropriate antibiotics. Adenomatous polyps may be removed by snare polypectomy during colonoscopy. Cancers and Meckel's diverticulum can be treated by resection of the relevant area of bowel (see Ch. 6). Small bowel ulceration resulting from NSAIDs is usually self-limiting, although severe cases may require surgery. Arteriovenous malformations (e.g. telangiectasia or angiodysplasia) may be treated by colonoscopic diathermy coagulation or laser photocoagulation. However, extensive lesions (especially in the right colon) are best treated by resection (Leicester 1990).

Patients presenting with lower GI bleeding, and their families, experience similar fears to those with upper GI bleeding. They may also have to face invasive procedures or surgery. The nurse needs to create a partnership with patients and their families. Through this, the nurse can establish a relationship of trust and reassurance, helping patients and their families to cope with the situation they are in and providing them with a central person to whom they may turn for support.

Angiography

Angiography can play a part in diagnosing and treating GI bleeding of arterio-capillary origin. However, it is generally limited to patients in whom other methods have failed to show the bleeding site or to stop it. The purpose of angiography in such cases should, according to Rossi & Pavone (1990), be to demonstrate the site of gastrointestinal bleeding and to perform a procedure which will provide definitive control of the bleeding – intra-arterial infusion of vasoconstricting drugs or transcatheter embolisation.

Intra-arterial infusion of vasoconstricting drugs, primarily vasopressin, may be used to control bleeding in all GI areas apart from the upper two-thirds of the oesophagus (this is because the direct aortic origin of the arterial branches supplying this area makes the procedure very difficult). It is important to monitor all patients receiving vasoconstricting drugs carefully for side-effects of general vasoconstriction. This procedure is used less frequently since, as mentioned, its value is debatable.

Percutaneous transcatheter embolisation of the bleeding site provides an alternative therapeutic approach for reduction and control of haemorrhage. Reabsorbable or non-reabsorbable materials are used for embolisation depending on the bleeding site and the underlying condition. The side of the vessel to be occluded also influences the type of material used.

Embolisation allows stabilisation of the patient's condition and, should surgery still be required, an elective operation can be performed with much less risk (Rossi & Pavone 1990). It may, however, prove the definitive treatment.

Angiography is sometimes helpful when diagnosing haemorrhage from lesions in the small intestine.

Psychological considerations

Virtually all patients who experience GI bleeding, be it upper or lower, will experience hospitalisation at some point, even if only as an outpatient.

In entering the patient role, an individual is placing himself in a position of both dependence and uncertainty. This role may not be welcomed by the patient or his family, and in such situations nurses are in a good position to act as the patient's advocate in ensuring that at the centre of the treatment is a person, not a list of symptoms – someone who has a right to information to make decisions about his own body and treatment. Thorough and continuous nursing assessment highlights the patient's position as a member of a wider group of family and friends and also highlights that, if the patient wishes, they too may need to be involved in discussions on treatment options.

Any sense of dependence and uncertainty that a patient feels may well be exaggerated by the potentially emotional atmosphere that surrounds disease. Some patients presenting with GI bleeding may eventually have to face diagnosis of a chronic or life-threatening condition, and they may also have to face the prospect of body-image-changing surgery or the need for major readjustments to their lifestyle.

Patients' worries may centre on financial concerns, as hospitalisation may mean loss of, or reduction in, income. They may relate to such concerns as body image, which O'Brien (1980) defined as 'interpersonal experience of our feelings and attitudes towards our bodies and the way we organise these experiences'. Wassner (1982) pointed out that our body image gives us a sense of existence, a basis for our identity, and goes on to state that: 'Changed body image may alter social responses and lead to stigmatisation and hence may diminish or destroy identity.'

Patients who experience GI bleeding may have to face a change in their body image for a wide variety of reasons. It may be the need for a stoma formation following bowel resection, or significant weight loss, or jaundice and caput medusae following liver failure, or scars following surgery. Whatever the reason for a change in body image, it creates the necessity for major readjustment in how patients (and those around them) perceive themselves.

The attitude of nurses and all health care professionals is vital in helping the patient and their family to cope. For some patients, the biggest challenge they will have to cope with is facing the uncertainty of their diagnosis and the very common fear of cancer. For some people, the concern about cancer may override everything else, and may impair their ability to assimilate information.

Depression, described by Orr (1987) as 'a profound state which is characterised by feelings of loss, low self esteem, worthlessness, shame ... or hopelessness', may also affect many patients presenting with GI bleeds. It may simply be the fact that they are ill and separated from loved ones, or that they are facing a life-threatening illness or a chronic condition. Whatever the situation, depression, if unresolved, may lead to a further impairment of physical health (Wassner 1982). Leidy et al (1990) pointed out that, usually, the most people want is a good quality of life with feelings of well-being and opportunities for personal development. They reinforce the fact that nurses are in a prime position, along with the rest of the clinical team, to support and assist those with chronic physical illness to achieve the best possible quality of life.

Watts (1991) highlighted the way in which nurses are best positioned to consider the interrelationships between the environment, the patient and their appraisal of their situation. Without recognising these links through assessment of clients, nurses cannot achieve the best for their patients. It may be through contacting social services to improve domestic arrangements for a patient at home, or it may be by talking to patients about their lifestyle and socialising habits, to enable them to envisage, for example, a life without alcohol.

Whatever nurses do, it is important to recognise that they have an invaluable contribution to make in enabling patients, including those with GI bleeding to, 'restore, maintain or enhance their health and assist them in fulfilling their potential' (Leidy et al 1990) for however long or short their life.

With this in mind, nursing assessments need to be holistic and comprehensive, emphasising the individualised nature of patient care. They will lead to a greater and more effective therapeutic relationship. They will enable the nurse to help alleviate the anxieties of the patients, their families and friends, and will assist the nurse to facilitate involvement of family and friends in support of the patient.

The value of this approach will be evident when greater patient understanding, reassurance and compliance with treatment is achieved. An individualised, patient-centred approach to care creates an environment in which nurses can maximise their role as the patient's advocate.

REFERENCES

Allan R, Dykes O 1976 A study of the factors influencing mortality rates from gastrointestinal haemorrhage. Quarterly Journal of Medicine 45:533–555
Burkitt H G, Quick C R G, Gatt D 1990 Essential surgery. Churchill Livingstone, London
Cutler J A Mendeloff A I 1981 Upper gastrointestinal bleeding, nature and magnitude of the problem in the U.S. Gastrointestinal Endoscopy 26(Suppl.):90
Graham D Y I 1991 Helicobacter pylori: its epidemiology and its role in duodenal ulcer disease. Journal of Gastroenterology and Hepatology 6:97
Graham D Y I, Malaty H M, Evans D G, Evans D I, Jr, Klein P D, Adam E 1991 Epidemiology of Helicobacter pylori in an asymptomatic population in the United States. Effect of age, race and socioeconomic status. Gastroenterology 100:1495
Hayes P C 1995 Editorial, portal hypertensive revisited. Quarterly Journal of Medicine 88:751–754
Holman R A E, Gough K R, Gartell P, Britton D C, Smith R B 1990 Value of a centralised approach in the management of haematemesis and melaena: experience in a district general hospital. Gut 31:504–508
Hunt P S et al 1979 Mortality in patients with haematemesis and melaena: a prospective study. British Medical Journal 1:1238–1240
Kumar P J, Clark M L (eds) 1989 Clinical medicine. Baillière Tindall, London
Lanza F L, Aspinall R L, Swabb E A, Davis R E, Rack M F, Rubin A 1989 Double-blind, placebo controlled endoscopic comparison of the mucosal protective effects of misoprostol versus cimetidine or tolmetin-induced mucosal injury to the stomach and duodenum. Gastroenterology 95:289
Leicester R J 1990 Gastrointestinal haemorrhage. Medicine International 77, May:3188–3193
Leidy N K, Ozbolt J G, Swain M A P 1990 Psycho-psychological processes of stress in chronic physical illness: a theoretical perspective. Journal of Advanced Nursing 15:478–486
Malhotra S L 1978 A comparison of unrefined wheat and rice diets in the management of duodenal ulcers. Postgraduate Medicine Journal 54:6
Morris A I 1992 Upper gastrointestinal haemorrhage – endoscopic approaches to diagnosis and treatment. In: Gilmore I T, Shields R (eds) Gastrointestinal emergencies. W B Saunders, London
O'Brien J 1980 Mirror, mirror, why me? Nursing Mirror 150(17):36–37

Orr J (ed.) 1987 Women's health in the community. John Wiley, Sussex

Ovaska J T, Havia T 1988 Surgical treatment of high gastric ulcer. Annalles Chirurgiae et Gynaecologiae 77:6–8

Rossi P, Pavone P 1990 Upper gastrointestinal bleeding. In: Dondelinger R F, Rossi P, Kurdziel J C, Wallace S (eds) Interventional radiology. Theime Medical Publishers, New York

Shields R 1989 Variceal haemorrhage. Current Practice in Surgery 1(1):10–16

Shields R 1992 Bleeding oesaphageal varices. In: Gilmore I T, Shields R (eds) Gastrointestinal emergencies. W B Saunders, London

Sleisenger M H, Fordtran J S 1993 Gastrointestinal disease, vol 1. W B Saunders, Philadelphia

Snyman J H, Dykes P W, Keighley R M B 1992 Upper gastrointerstinal haemorrhage – overview of treatment. In: Gilmore I T, Shields R (eds) Gastrointestinal emergencies. W B Saunders, London

Spicer C C, Stewart D N, Winser D M de R 1944 Perforated peptic ulcer during the period of heavy air raids. Lancet 1:14

Stringer M D, Cameron A E P 1988 Surgeon's attitudes to the operative management of duodenal ulcer perforation and haemorrhage. Annals of the Royal College of Surgeons of England 70: 220–223

Taylor S, Chisholm G D, O'Higgins N, Shields R (eds) 1984 Surgical management. Heineman, London

Tennant C 1988 Psychological causes of duodenal ulcer. Australia and New Zealand Journal of Psychiatry 22:195

Travis S P L, Taylor R M, Misiewicz J J 1993 Gastroenterology. Blackwell Scientific, London

Wassner A 1982 The impact of mutilating surgery or trauma on body image. International Nursing Review 29(3):86–90

Watts M 1991 Psychology – themes in nursing. In: Perry A, Jolley M (eds) Nursing, a knowledge base for practice. Hodder and Stoughton, London

---

FURTHER READING

Edwards C R W, Bouchier I A D (eds) 1991 Davidson's principles and practice of medicine, 16th edn. Churchill Livingstone, London

Hayes P C, Redhead D N, Finlayson N D C 1994 Transjugular intrahepatic portosystemic stent shunts. Gut 35:445–446

Joffe S N 1989 Endoscopic laser control of gastrointestinal haemorrhage. Current Practice in Surgery 1(1):25–33

Snyman J H, Keighley R M B 1989 Acute non-variceal haemorrhage. Current Practice in Surgery 1(1):2–9

The acute abdomen

Wendy Atkin   Jill Calvert

■ **CONTENTS**

INTRODUCTION

Due to the complexity of this subject, the most frequently encountered conditions within the surgical gastrointestinal field will be considered and divided into two main headings:

- peritonitis
- obstruction.

Initially, common factors in patients presenting with an acute abdomen will be discussed, with particular emphasis on pain. Predisposing conditions of the upper gastrointestinal tract will then be detailed, followed by a case study. This is followed by conditions of the lower gut which lead to an acute abdomen.

Due to the acute onset and severity of symptoms which a patient with an acute abdomen can experience, hospital admission is inevitable and surgical intervention is often necessary. Many of the causes are serious and potentially life-threatening, and will require prompt and efficient treatment. Others may only become apparent after a period of observation and investigation.

As the patient's condition is potentially unstable and could rapidly become critical, nurses must be able to give immediate reactive management to actual problems and anticipate potential problems, which will preempt and initiate a proactive approach to care. The efficient management of the care given to a patient will be underpinned by the degree of expertise, knowledge and understanding of the primary named nurse (Alfaro 1990). A nurse specialising in gastroenterology will have the opportunity to develop the depth of knowledge and skills required to obtain and interpret essential information when making a nursing diagnosis within the assessment process. The efficiency and accuracy of this process will then be fundamental to the planning, implementation and evaluation of care, in order to achieve a successful outcome.

In spending more time with the patient than the examining doctor, nurses are able to contribute invaluable information by assessing physical signs and symptoms, as well as the psychological and sociological needs of the patient.

Pain is the characteristic feature of any patient presenting with an acute abdomen. An accurate assessment and history of the nature, type and location of the pain experienced is imperative, as detailed later in this chapter. Accompanying signs or symptoms of nausea, vomiting, altered bowel habit, anorexia and fever, and the patient's past medical history and lifestyle all contribute towards the assessment.

The main complications associated with an acute abdomen are shock, peritonitis and haemorrhage (see Ch. 5 for haemorrhage). It is essential that any patient admitted with an acute abdomen receives prompt attention, so that their symptoms may be best alleviated, and the risk of complications minimised.

INITIAL OBSERVATIONS OF THE PRESENTING PATIENT

Initial observations provide an assessment on which to base decisions about the condition and care of the patient. Patients will usually present with severe abdominal pain, which is frequently associated with vomiting. The nurse's priority is to promote the patient's comfort by identifying and offering appropriate symptom relief in collaboration with the medical staff.

GENERAL NURSING CARE OF A PATIENT PRESENTING WITH ACUTE ABDOMINAL PAIN

Acute abdominal pain may be caused by inflammation, ischaemia, spasm, or irritation of the serous membranes.

Pain is often the initial symptom or warning sign that stimulates the patient to seek medical advice. Pain will have degrees of severity and the patient may have been suffering for hours or days. The patient's response to the pain is usually of a protective nature. The character and perception of the pain and the patient's response to it will be unique to each individual, and is known to be dependent on past experiences, beliefs held, culture and anxiety levels (Hayward 1975, Gibson 1994).

Assessment

The nurse's possession of good observational and communication skills is important. The site, duration, character, radiation and exacerbating or relieving factors will all help to determine the cause of the pain. The information available can be enhanced by pain assessment tools, including visual analogue scales, which may be useful in helping to ensure that all patients, regardless of personality or the response to their pain, receive adequate analgesia. Such assessment tools can serve to increase the patient's involvement in their care. This approach, coupled with an individual care system such as primary nursing, helps to build a therapeutic relationship between the nurse and the patient. Pain relief may then be discussed between them and treatment can be evaluated effectively.

Location

The patient may not be able to define the precise whereabouts of the source of pain they are experiencing. This is due to the close proximity of the abdominal organs' sensory representation in the brain. Pain may be described as dull, diffuse, deep-seated or generalised, making it difficult to pinpoint. It may appear to move from one area to another or be referred pain.

The perception of abdominal pain is mediated by the autonomic nervous system and is often referred to as visceral pain, which is within the abdomen. Pain at the surface/skin level arises from the stimulations of visceral nerve endings in the corresponding skin dermatomes of the affected abdominal organ. These pass along the path of the sympathetic nerves, to enter the lumbar (L1-2) or thoracic (T6–12) regions of the spinal cord.

A useful way to describe the locality is to divide the abdomen into quarters, with a central region. There may be a correlation between locality and cause, but this is frequently not the case.

Severity

It was suggested by Bond & Pearson (1969) and Griffiths (1980) that patients with extrovert personalities were more likely to express the severity of their pain and receive analgesia than were introverts. However, they may be perceived by health care professionals as demanding, whilst introverts are seen as stoic people. Categorising patients thus is not helpful, and as the sensation of pain is subjective, it is here that pain assessment tools may be useful. Tools in an acute setting need to be simple and easy to use, requiring minimal explanation and effort to be effective.

Character

Pain can be described by the patient as spasmodic, sharp, dragging, heavy/crushing or hot/burning. The pain induced by distension or excessive contraction from a hollow viscus, such as that due to obstruction of the intestine or gall bladder, causes the patient to experience bouts of excruciating spasmodic pain or colic. This is due to increased muscle contraction in an attempt to push contents past the obstruction.

Pain may also be due to the process of inflammation. Heat and swelling will sensitise the nerve endings. The oedema and vascular congestion that accompanies the inflammation causes stretching of the gut which activates the pain receptors.

An understanding of the type of pain will greatly influence the analgesia given. Correlating the pharmacological effects of different drugs with the cause of the pain will give greater efficacy, e.g. non-steroidal anti-inflammatory agents such as diclofenac sodium for inflammatory pain, opiates (including morphine or pethidine) for more severe pain, or using combinations of analgesics for optimum effect.

Duration

The duration of pain is a very important factor in determining its cause. When the pain started and for how long it was experienced at particular levels should be ascertained. The pattern of pain experienced, i.e. whether it is constant or intermittent, should also be noted.

Exacerbating factors

Is the pain worse on movement – particularly movement of the abdomen, on deep breathing or coughing? Is the pain stimulated by eating certain foods, or due to the increase in peristalsis by eating?

Relieving factors

Information needs to be gained about what, other than analgesia, makes the pain more tolerable – lying still, certain body posture such as flexing knees, holding the affected part, guarding, vomiting or defaecation?

A general assessment of the patient is imperative, including facial expression, mood, body posture, skin colour and pallor – is there any sweating or clamminess? Consideration should be given to what is being communicated verbally and non-verbally. Baseline measurements of blood pressure, pulse, respiratory rate and temperature are required. Initially, pain will cause tachycardia and hypertension from sympathetic overactivity. This cardiovascular response may disguise some of the symptoms of hypovolaemia. However, the body cannot maintain these physiological or behavioural manifestations and, as the duration of the pain extends, adaptation takes place, and physiological responses to shock override those to pain, even though the pain may still be experienced (McCaffrey 1972).

Management of pain

Any patient in acute abdominal pain will probably be frightened and anxious, making the management of pain a complex issue. No one factor will ensure comfort alone. Several strategies and combinations of pain-relieving factors will need to be utilised.

The management of pain is split into pharmacological and non-pharmacological measures. When there is a possibility of analgesia masking symptoms, which requires delayed assessment, nurses and medical staff should collaborate together and with the patient in choosing and timing the administration of drugs. Patients should not be left in pain waiting for a doctor to examine them.

Depending on the nature and severity of the pain, analgesia may be considered, such as anti-inflammatory medication in conjunction with an opiate. The appropriate administrative route will depend on the severity of the pain, the drug, the acceptability to the patient and the patient's existing or previous medical history.

Complementary to analgesics are non-analgesic approaches to the relief of pain. These include:

- communication and provision of information to reduce anxiety levels
- distraction
- careful handling, support and positioning of the patient
- appropriate use of touch, presence of nursing staff, or relatives when so desired by the patient
- massage, relaxation and deep breathing
- imagery may also have a role in acute pain, especially if used to aid a patient through a particularly uncomfortable procedure / examination.

For pain relief to be effective the nurse needs to address the physical and psychological needs of the patient. The value of the nurse's presence, advising and teaching techniques such as imagery, distraction and relaxation can be particularly helpful. This can also be an opportunity for patients to talk about themselves and their presenting illness and for the nurse to give explanations of their care and likely interventions during their admission (Mobily et al 1993).

Evaluation of pain relief is continuous in the acute phase. This evaluation should be by the patient. After all, it is their pain. While recognising the value of enabling patients to retain some control, the nurse remains the patient's advocate throughout. It is the authors' experience that an effective therapeutic nurse / patient relationship, and the subsequent reduction of anxiety levels in patients, leads to a reduction in the required amounts of analgesia.

SHOCK

Shock occurs when the cardiovascular system fails to deliver adequate oxygen and nutrients to meet the metabolic needs of the body. This may be due to à decreased circulating blood volume, as a result of either haemorrhage or an excessive fluid loss such as that incurred by vomiting or diarrhoea. Alternatively, it can be due to dilatation of the vascular system stimulated by chemical responses to infection or toxins.

Septic shock may also arise from acute gastrointestinal problems. This results in tissue damage caused by the chemicals produced in the inflammatory response to bacteria. As the toxins interact with cell membranes, the inflammatory response is activated, chemicals are produced, cells are damaged and vasodilation occurs. The damage incurred can lead to respiratory, renal or cardiac failure.

The signs and symptoms of shock will vary depending on the severity of the condition. The primary characteristics of shock include:

1. Hypotension, systolic blood pressure (BP) lower than 95 mmHg. This is a result of generalised vasodilation. (Once the BP falls below 60 mmHg the perfusion pressure through the coronary arteries may be insufficient and the myocardium becomes ischaemic. The patient will feel dizzy and vague and is likely to be anxious.
2. Pulse will be weak and rapid (over 100 beats / min) in an effort to increase cardiac output.

3. The skin will be pale, clammy and cool due to vasoconstriction of peripheral blood vessels.
4. Sweating will occur due to sympathetic nervous system stimulation and increased levels of adrenaline.
5. Oliguria results from hypotension as levels of aldosterone and antidiuretic hormone are raised to increase water reabsorption. Dehydration occurs when the patient has been prevented from taking anything orally due to pain, coupled with excessive fluid loss by vomiting and diarrhoea. Dehydration may be indicated by loss of skin turgour, furred tongue and, in later stages, sunken eyes.
6. Patients experience thirst, because osmoreceptors sense increased blood concentration and trigger the thirst sensation from the hypothalamus.
7. Acidosis occurs due to metabolic dysfunction, causing a build-up of lactic acid.

When the body can no longer compensate for the low blood volume, irreversible shock results. Prolonged underperfusion of any organ leads to cellular anoxia and tissue death, ultimately leading to the death of the patient. Once a patient is in irreversible shock, intervention will not save them.

PERITONITIS

Peritonitis is inflammation of the peritoneal cavity, which includes the serosal covering of the bowel, mesentery, omentum and the lining of the abdominal cavity. The inflammation is usually in response to bacterial invasion or chemical irritation from bile, urine, or pancreatic, gastric or intestinal secretions, which have leaked into the peritoneal cavity.

Primary infective peritonitis is usually due to *Escherichia coli*, but may also present as a mixed flora including *Clostridium*, *Klebsiella*, *Pseudomonas*, and *Bacteroides*. Secondary peritonitis is most commonly seen in surgical patients, but may also occur following a stab wound or traumatic injury, resulting in perforation of the intestinal tract.

Peritonitis may be either localised or generalised:

- Localised peritonitis
    - appendicitis
    - cholecystitis
    - pancreatitis
    - diverticulitis
    - pylonephritis
    - cystitis

- Generalised peritonitis
    - duodenal ulcer
    - gastric ulcer
    - appendicitis
    - diverticulitis
    - abdominal surgery.

Localised peritonitis involves the transmural inflammation of the bowel, as seen in appendicitis and diverticulitis, or it may progress into general peritonitis. Acute peritonitis may also lead to a paralysis of the intestinal tract (paralytic ileus) and later to adhesions and mechanical obstruction of the bowel.

Generalised peritonitis, if untreated, is life-threatening. This is due to shock caused by the gross exudation of fluid in response to inflammation which leads to hypovolaemia. This will be further complicated by the development of toxaemia from the absorbed toxic metabolites or septicaemia if there is infection present.

Specific features of peritonitis

The patient will usually describe abdominal pain as constant, diffuse and intense. The abdomen will become distended by gas and fluid in the intestine and later by the escape of fluid into the peritoneal cavity. Examination of the abdomen needs to be gentle as the patient will experience extreme rebound tenderness and may be rigid with guarding. Guarding is an involuntary spasm of the abdominal wall indicating peritonitis. This may be localised to one area or may be generalised over the whole abdomen.

Rebound tenderness occurs when sharp pain is experienced as the hand is removed suddenly from the abdomen due to the sudden movement of the inflamed peritoneum.

Bowel sounds are decreased or absent, due to paralytic ileus. The patient may not have had a bowel movement for some days. The patient may be nauseated and vomiting due to metabolic disturbance, obstruction or pain.

The patient may be feverish, as pyrexia occurs with infection and inflammation (associated with a raised leucocyte count above $11\,000/mm^3$).

Tachycardia occurs to compensate for the decrease in blood volume, as well as being a result of raised metabolic rate in the presence of pyrexia. Respirations may be shallow and rapid as a result of acidosis, pain, shock and compression from the distended abdomen.

Complications of peritonitis

An intraperitoneal abscess may form as a result of the pus collection within the omental walls of the peritoneal cavity. The pus often gravitates to the pelvis, causing pelvic abscesses. They may also form in the subphrenic and subhepatic spaces and between loops of bowel. If peritonitis remains untreated, the accumulation of fluid in the bowel leads to further dilatation, the patient becomes increasingly dehydrated and toxic, and vomiting becomes more profuse and consists of small bowel contents. The pulse progressively becomes weak and rapid, as hypovolaemia, sepsis and shock supervene.

INVESTIGATIONS

Investigations a patient may undergo will include:

1. full blood count for anaemia or raised white cell count indicating response to infection

2. serum urea and electrolytes may indicate dehydration, renal impairment and deranged electrolyte levels
3. serum amylase levels may be elevated in any acute abdominal condition; if elevated greater than five times the normal, this indicates acute pancreatitis
4. serum for blood grouping and cross-matching will be taken in preparation for transfusion if surgery is required
5. arterial blood gases and pH should be evaluated if the patient is in shock or has a history of respiratory disease
6. erect chest X-ray and supine X-ray of the abdomen will detect air under the diaphragm which indicates perforation; dilated loops of bowel or fluid levels are suggestive of obstruction
7. ultrasound scanning may identify calculi or fluid collections.

COMMUNICATION

It is essential that the patient has the opportunity to express concerns and anxieties on admission to the ward. As Bailey & Clark (1991) identified, anxiety is a result of the threat experienced by an individual due to a hospital admission and/or presence of illness. Therefore, good communication skills are imperative to identify and alleviate anxiety. The availability of one identified nurse as a named or primary nurse will greatly facilitate the development of a therapeutic relationship. Within a short period of time, mutual trust and respect may be gained to promote and achieve efficacy in meeting a patient's needs. Additional communication with the patient's family and partners will help to allay their fears and anxieties, providing them with essential support.

AN ACUTE ABDOMEN ASSOCIATED WITH UPPER GASTROINTESTINAL TRACT PATHOLOGY

Some of the specific causes of an acute abdomen associated with upper GI tract pathology are detailed below.

Peptic ulceration

Peptic ulceration is the collective term for ulceration in the upper GI tract where pepsin is secreted. A peptic ulcer is an erosion found in the mucosal wall of the stomach, pylorus or duodenum. Erosion is caused by excess secretion of hydrochloric acid in relation to the amount of mucus secreted and reduced neutralisation of gastric acid by the duodenal, biliary and pancreatic fluids. Peptic ulceration is believed to be due to a defective mucosal defence, as ulceration does not occur in the absence of acid and pepsin secretion (Forrest et al 1991). *Helicobacter pylori* is thought to cause most peptic ulceration, and suggested treatment includes antibiotics and protein pump inhibitors such as Omeprazole.

Perforated peptic ulcer

This is perforation caused by the ulcer eroding the wall of the stomach or duodenum. Gastric contents or bile escape into the peritoneal cavity, causing a chemical and then a bacterial peritonitis.

Distinguishing features
- Pain – severe and constant, usually of sudden onset in epigastrium often exacerbated by movement; on examination the abdomen is very tender and there is intense guarding
- vomiting – vomit will be brownish or blood-stained
- tachycardia
- pyrexial
- respiration is usually shallow.

Most of these features are characteristic of peritonitis, whatever the cause.

Investigations
Usually diagnosis can be made on the symptoms alone. Erect chest X-ray will usually reveal gas under the diaphragm.

Specific care
The patient will require preparation for emergency surgery if perforation is suspected. The nature of surgery will depend on the location of the perforated ulcer and the patient's past medical history. In the case of a perforated gastric ulcer, a partial gastrectomy may be performed to resect the whole ulcer. Vagotomy and pyloroplasty may be performed if there is a past medical history of treated peptic ulcers (see Ch. 5). A perforated duodenal ulcer will be oversewn.

Acute cholecystitis
Acute inflammation of the gall bladder is commonly caused by the obstruction of the cystic duct by a small stone, with proximal distention of the gall bladder and secondary infection.

Specific symptoms
The patient will be tender in the right upper quadrant, pain being exacerbated on inspiration. The patient will also have a fever and tachycardia, owing to the systemic response to the inflamed, obstructed gall bladder. Symptoms will persist over several days before subsiding.

Biliary colic
Spasm of the smooth muscle in the cystic duct is caused by its obstruction by a stone.

Specific symptoms
The pain these patients experience is severe, reaching a peak in the first minutes after onset and continuing for hours or until an opiate is given. Symptoms should resolve within hours. No fever is experienced and there is often a history of similar episodes.

Acute pancreatitis
Acute pancreatitis is a potentially life-threatening illness, ultimately affecting

every system of the body in severe cases. It is thought to occur as a result of obstruction of the drainage of the exocrine pancreas, either by calculi from the bile-ducts or persistent excessive alcohol intake. In the latter, mucous plugs may develop in pancreatic drainage ducts and the tone of the sphincter of Oddi is increased, inhibiting enzyme drainage. Alcohol or the presence of bile in pancreatic ducts stimulates enzyme production and activation, and thus the inflammation and oedema associated with pancreatitis commence. The illness can become protracted when complications arise, resulting in a long hospital admission. Only occasionally is surgical intervention indicated.

Usually, the patient's symptoms are treated with aggressive fluid and colloid replacement regimes and analgesia. The patient's condition is monitored and repeated reassessment of their responses is undertaken. Caring for a patient with acute pancreatitis presents a tremendous nursing challenge. It is the nurse who monitors the patient's condition, observing for the early signs of complications while relieving the pain and anxiety caused by the illness. Acute pancreatitis is frightening for the patient and the intensity of care given may heighten anxiety about the potential seriousness of their condition.

Patients with pancreatitis almost always present with epigastric pain, and their symptoms are usually similar to cholecystitis initially (cholecystitis may coexist). The majority of patients will have a mild or moderate degree of pancreatitis and recover without complication. For a few, deterioration to a severe form of acute pancreatitis can be rapid, and in necrotising haemorrhagic pancreatitis, mortality is high. Hence the team involved in caring for a person with acute pancreatitis will need to gather accurate data from monitoring the patient's condition and respond appropriately. It is the need for constant monitoring and vigilance which may concern patients or their families.

Patients who do develop severe pancreatitis are at particular risk of death, because the breakdown of the pancreas and surrounding structures causes overwhelming toxaemia and adult respiratory distress syndrome. Severe fluid loss to the abdomen disrupts fluid balance and induces shock. Electrolyte imbalance and hypocalcaemia further disturb homeostatic mechanisms, and the patient requires intensive therapy support. In addition to the nurse's close observation of the patient's vital signs, fluid balance and pain, daily blood tests will be required, in order to check:

- haemoglobin and white cell count – indicate haemorrhage and inflammatory response
- arterial blood gas estimations – indicate respiratory and metabolic impairment
- blood glucose levels – indicate damage to endocrine pancreas
- serum amylase levels – five times greater than normal indicates acute pancreatitis
- urea, electrolyte, calcium and phosphate levels – indicate fluid and electrolyte disturbance associated with tissue damage
- liver function tests – indicate enzyme levels and degree of pancreatic damage.

Discharge arrangements should be considered as soon as the patient's condition is stable, to ensure that adequate support at home is arranged. Returning home is very daunting for the patient and their family after such an illness. After a long stay in the safe, secure environment of the hospital, with all of the professional care readily available, it can be disconcerting for patients to have it suddenly withdrawn. The long-term implications of the illness for lifestyle, diet and alcohol consumption need to be discussed with the patient and the family. Once feelings of guilt and self-blame have been addressed, ongoing support and counselling may be required, particularly if the pancreatitis was caused by a high alcohol intake. The principles underpinning the care associated with acute pancreatitis are illustrated in Case history 6.1.

Case history 6.1   Pancreatitis: a nursing challenge

Ann, a 55-year-old retired nurse, was admitted to hospital experiencing severe epigastric pain, nausea and vomiting. A diagnosis of pancreatitis secondary to alcohol intake was made, when ultrasound scan showed no evidence of gallstones, and was coupled with a significantly raised serum amylase. Ann reported that she was a regular party-goer, consuming more than 40 units of alcohol a week. Ann was accompanied by her partner David, who subsequently proved to be a great source of support and comfort to her.

On first meeting Ann, she was frightened and restless, and her facial expression and shallow breathing indicated she was experiencing considerable pain.

Ann's pain was assessed, and the site and severity were noted. Ann described her pain as excruciating, which was corroborated by her rapid and shallow breathing pattern – deep breathing obviously exacerbated her pain. Ann was helped to find the position that was for her most comfortable and analgesia was administered. As morphine is thought to stimulate contraction of the sphincter of Oddi, leading to increased pain, pethidine was administered (Kumar & Clark 1994).

Explanations about her condition, and David's presence, helped Ann to relax, giving the analgesia an opportunity to take effect. When Ann realised that her pain would be reviewed regularly, she began to appear less anxious. Ann clearly found having the same nurse caring for her reassuring, and a trusting relationship was quickly established. By maintaining continuity, assessments of her general condition and pain were considered to be more reliable. Any increased intensity in the pain she was experiencing, coupled with growing abdominal distension, would be early indicators of complications such as obstruction, formation of subphrenic and/or subhepatic abscesses or haemorrhage.

Because of the diagnosis of pancreatitis, further assessment of her respiratory function was indicated. There was a real threat of adult respiratory distress due to shock and inadequate gaseous exchange as a result of reduced production of surfactant in the alveoli of the lungs. The rate and depth of breathing and the colour of her skin were noted. Measurement of her oxygen saturations and her rapid shallow breathing revealed a need for humidified oxygen therapy. The face mask coupled with the noise from the humidifier

Case history 6.1 *(cont'd)*

made communication very difficult – she was becoming frightened again. However, with David's constant presence and the obvious experience of her nurse, Ann began to feel safer.

Initially it was assumed that, as Ann was a retired nurse, she would have some knowledge of pancreatitis and its implications. This was found not to be the case and raised an important point. Patients' knowledge should not be assumed by those caring for them; their understanding should be clarified when information is given. Subsequently, less technical explanations resulted in a better understanding of what was happening to her.

Her cardiovascular status was assessed and monitored regularly, looking for signs of hypovolaemia, haemorrhage and sepsis. An inflamed pancreas can haemorrhage if the blood vessels become eroded by the autodigestion of the pancreatic tissue. Sepsis can then occur. Evaluation of blood pressure and heart rate together with Ann's overall appearance, skin temperature and colour were made. Any reports of dizziness and vagueness from Ann would be regarded as suspicious.

Ann's fluid status needed careful monitoring; the need for a urinary catheter was explained to Ann. By ensuring adequate explanations and privacy for Ann during this procedure, the potential embarrassment was minimised.

A central venous line was also inserted to monitor Ann's circulating venous pressure. The frequency and intensity of Ann's care resulted in her having little time to rest. No sooner had she been assisted to get comfortable than she needed to be disturbed again. Ann was becoming exhausted by the never-ending round of observations. Consequently, a specific rest period was negotiated whereby no one disturbed her.

It was explained to Ann that surgery was not indicated; her treatment would be supportive in nature, giving time for the inflammation to resolve spontaneously.

Measures to 'rest' the pancreas and reduce pancreatic activity were explained to Ann. This involved nasogastric intubation to drain gastric secretions, which would prevent gastric acid from entering the duodenum thus reducing the stimulation to release gastric hormones such as secretin and cholecystokinin-pancreozymin. Ann was asked not to eat or drink anything, to reduce the production of pancreatic enzymes. When the pancreatic ducts become obstructed, there may be retrograde flow of bile into the ducts, stimulating the production of enzymes and resulting in autodigestion. Enzymes and blood may escape into the peritoneal cavity causing pseudocysts (pseudocysts are an accumulation of exudating pancreatic tissue which have become encapsulated by fibrous tissue, but have no epithelial lining), peritonitis, paralytic ileus or obstruction caused by pressure of the swollen pancreas on the duodenum.

Ann found her nasogastric tube extremely uncomfortable, as her nose and throat became sore. The trauma was reduced by carefully securing the tube. Her mouth became quite dry despite rehydration with intravenous fluids. Regular mouthwashes and lipsalve helped relieve these intensely uncomfortable symptoms. Her fluid status was regularly evaluated, with fluids given being carefully titrated to replace losses.

Parenteral nutrition would be indicated if her condition did not resolve within a few days, since malnutrition would then be a possibility.

Case history 6.1 *(cont'd)*

Alpha and beta cells found in the islets of Langerhans in the pancreas control blood glucose levels. The alpha cells secrete glucagon, which is needed for the conversion of glycogen in the liver to glucose (glycogenolysis) and for the conversion of amino acids, glycerol and lactic acid to glucose (gluconeogenesis). This glucose is released into the bloodstream and raises the glucose levels. The beta cells produce insulin which is needed to transport the glucose from the blood into the cells. The potential for deranged blood glucose levels was high. It was explained to Ann why blood levels needed to be checked frequently, and when they became unstable insulin was administered. Strict rotation of puncture sites for capillary blood testing reduced some of Ann's dread of having this done, but her fingers still became sore. Ann was feeling decidedly battered and bruised by this time.

Obstruction of the common bile duct resulted in jaundice; the intense itchiness of Ann's skin could only be relieved by cool sponging and the application of calamine lotion. Her anxiety was relieved by careful explanations and constant reassurance that it would resolve when her condition abated. Due to increased bilirubin, her urine was much darker in colour, and her stools became pale as a result of reduced urobilinogen. Assessment of bowel movements and the passage of flatus was undertaken, as these would indicate resumption of peristaltic activity.

Ann's progress was seriously complicated by the formation of infected pseudocysts (abscesses). These were managed with antibiotics, and Ann had to endure having a 'pigtail' drain inserted under CT guidance. The pseudocysts resulted in continuing pain for Ann.

Despite the intense nursing care Ann received, her condition suddenly deteriorated. Displaying signs of shock, she had developed septicaemia due to the abscesses and peritonitis. Emergency intervention to resuscitate her was instigated. The seriousness of her condition was carefully explained to David by the primary nurse and doctor. David received frequent and regular reports of Ann's condition in an effort to support and comfort him. However, Ann suffered a fatal respiratory arrest, and David was naturally devastated. He continues to visit Ann's nurses, reinforcing the concept that a therapeutic relationship had been formed and maintained which enabled David to feel comfortable about returning to the place where Ann had died. His care continues with ongoing support from a bereavement group.

AN ACUTE ABDOMEN ASSOCIATED WITH LOWER GASTROINTESTINAL TRACT PATHOLOGY

Some of the specific causes of an acute abdomen associated with lower GI tract pathology are detailed below.

Acute appendicitis

Acute appendicitis is an inflammation of the appendix due to infection. This may be due to an obstruction and invasion by *Escherichia coli* or anaerobes, caecal carcinoma in the elderly, or Crohn's disease. It occurs most frequently in young adults in developed countries.

Distinguishing features

- Abdominal pain – the classical diagnostic symptom of pain is that it begins in the mid-abdomen as a vague central abdominal pain, and after a varying period (hours to 2–3 days) the pain intensifies and localises in the right lower quadrant. However, only approximately one-half of the patients with appendicitis will present in this way. The remaining patients will present with a variety of patterns of pain.
- Temperature – the skin may often feel hot to touch, but the patient may not always be pyrexial. The while blood cell count may reveal a moderate leucocytosis.
- Nausea or vomiting and anorexia.
- Change in bowel habit (tendency to constipation).

Complications

- Subacute obstruction may occur in the elderly
- Perforation leading to peritonitis
- Surgery will be indicated in cases of acute abdominal pain with peritonitis.

Specific pre-operative care

- Evaluate vital signs to assess progression of infection
- Heat should not be applied over the area of pain, as there is the possibility of causing rupture of the appendix and peritonitis
- Aperients should not be administered as induced peristalsis may cause a perforation.

Postoperative care

- Pain relief
- Diet and fluids can be reintroduced as tolerated, if a straightforward appendicectomy has been performed, in conjunction with the surgical team's assessment of the patient's recovery
- The patient should get up and out of bed as soon as possible.

Intestinal obstruction

Intestinal obstruction can be found in the small or large bowel and can be classified as mechanical or non-mechanical obstruction.

Most intestinal obstruction is due to a mechanical blockage. Obstruction of the bowel leads to distension above the blockage, with increased secretion of fluid into the bowel. Bacterial translocation can occur from the distended stagnant bowel, causing septicaemia and pneumonia. If strangulation occurs, the blood supply is impeded leading to necrosis, perforation and peritonitis unless urgent treatment of the condition is undertaken.

Mechanical causes

These include:

- adhesions – resulting from previous surgery, inflammatory disease or abdominal sepsis
- malignancy

- bowel strangulation – volvulus (twisting of intestine)
- hernias
- bolus obstruction (impacted faeces or foreign bodies).

Complete obstruction of the small bowel will lead to proximal dilatation of the bowel. This will interrupt peristalsis and result in vomiting of the large volume of gastric, biliary and pancreatic secretions. The higher up the small bowel the obstruction occurs, the more immediate is the onset of vomiting. The nature of the vomit will give clues as to the level of obstruction. If there is partially digested food seen, it is likely to be a gastric outlet obstruction. Large volume vomits of bile indicate a reasonably proximal small bowel obstruction, while if the vomit is faecal, then it is likely that the obstruction is in the distal ileum or large bowel and has been present for a considerable time (days/weeks). Pain tends to be 'colicky' or cramping, and is not necessarily severe.

In large bowel obstruction, symptoms will develop more gradually, due to the ability of the colon and caecum to distend. Perforation may occur as the thin-walled caecum progressively distends. If the ileocaecal valve becomes incompetent (as in half of the cases of obstruction), this will allow the small bowel to distend and hence delay further the onset of symptoms. Distal to the obstruction, peristalsis ceases, gas is absorbed and *nothing* is passed per rectum.

If an obstruction is only partial or intermittent, symptoms will be erratic, with some vomiting but intermittent bowel action, for example. Furthermore, peristalsis will continue and be responsible for episodes of colicky pain. Peristaltic waves may even be visible over the abdomen – an effort to move gut contents past the obstruction.

In addition to a distended abdomen, increased bowel sounds, often high-pitched (tinkling), will be audible, owing to the increased peristaltic activity to that point. Absent bowel sounds suggest peritoneal involvement (peritonitis), in addition to the complete obstruction as seen in intestinal ischaemia or a strangulated bowel.

Adynamic bowel obstruction (paralytic ileus)

Paralytic ileus is non-mechanical obstruction due to a temporary disruption of the normal peristaltic activity, most commonly seen after abdominal surgery when the bowel has been handled.

Within the small bowel, this type of obstruction, referred to as paralytic ileus is usually seen postoperatively and lasts for up to 4 days. A more persistent 'ileus' may be due to postoperative complications such as an anastomotic leak, intra-abdominal infection, secondary to hypokalamia, or as a side-effect of some drug therapies.

In the large bowel, an adynamic obstruction may be caused by seemingly unrelated conditions, such as intra-abdominal inflammation or haemorrhage, pregnancy, multiple trauma or long-term immobility, and is referred to as pseudo-obstruction.

Distinguishing features

1. *Pain* will be caused by the proximal distension of the bowel with fluid and

swallowed air. The site of the pain experienced by the patient will often give an indication of the origin of the affected bowel. The patient may report the pain as varying in intensity and describe it as colicky in nature. This colic-type pain is caused by the increased peristalsis trying to pass the obstruction. If strangulation occurs the pain becomes continuous.

2. *Abdominal distension* observed in the patient may be caused by gas-filled loops of bowel. The lower down the gut the obstruction, the greater the distension.

3. *Vomiting* will be experienced by the patient if the obstruction is in the upper gut. If the vomiting is profuse, containing semidigested food, this would be suggestive of gastric outlet obstruction. When the patient has profuse vomiting of bile-stained fluid, upper small bowel obstruction would be suspected.

   Patients with lower bowel obstruction may not experience any vomiting. If vomiting does occur, the vomitus may be thick and 'faeculent', due to bacterial overgrowth in the static bowel contents. This is extremely unpleasant and alarming for the patient. Regardless of cause, measures to control the vomiting need to be taken, as excessive vomiting and lack of oral fluid intake will lead to dehydration and serum electrolyte imbalance. Mouth and lipcare for the patient should be freely available to refresh the mouth and alleviate the foul taste after each episode of vomiting.

4. *Altered bowel habit* – constipation and absence of the passage of flatus will occur as the movement of faeces is prevented distally to the obstruction and all bowel gas is absorbed. Therefore, a careful history and assessment of usual and recent bowel habits need to be made. For patients with subacute obstruction, the history may reveal a history of constipation alternating with diarrhoea. If the patient has a paralytic ileus, bowel sounds are often inaudible and the patient may not have passed anything rectally for some time.

5. *Anorexia* and dehydration may be experienced, as the patient is often afraid to eat or drink because this may exacerbate their vomiting and pain.

On examining the patient's abdomen there may be surprisingly little tenderness, except when strangulation has occurred. This requires immediate surgery.

Specific management

- Insertion of a nasogastric tube to decompress the bowel and relieve nausea and vomiting
- Intravenous infusion to replace fluid loss and to replenish serum electrolytes
- Assessment of the patient for surgery – some patients, such as those with Crohn's disease, who have frequent episodes of subacute intestinal obstruction may be managed conservatively initially
- Large bowel obstruction due to faecal impaction may be relieved by enemas
- Adynamic bowel obstruction usually resolves with conservative measures.

Surgery to remove the obstruction may be indicated. If strangulation can be excluded and the caecum is not dangerously distended, an operation can be deferred for a couple of days until the patient's condition is stable.

Strangulation of the bowel

This occurs when a segment of bowel becomes trapped, obstructing the lumen and disrupting the blood supply. If this is not relieved, infarction and perforation are probable. The main causes of a strangulated bowel are hernias, volvulus (rotation and twisting of the bowel) or adhesions.

The process of strangulation starts with partial obstruction of the bowel due to an external pressure or twisting, which leads to oedema of the bowel wall which in turn prevents venous return. As the obstruction progresses, the closed loop of bowel becomes increasingly dilated by gas fermentation. This combination of gas pressure and venous back-pressure inhibits arterial inflow, causing ischaemia and then infarction.

In the case of herniation, the bowel can become necrotic and perforate within the hernial sac, progressing to generalised peritonitis. A loop of bowel may become strangulated within the abdominal cavity if it becomes trapped by adhesions.

Volvulus

A volvulus is most commonly seen in the sigmoid colon, and is caused by chronic constipation.

Specific management of a sigmoid colon volvulus

A rectal tube to unkink and decompress the bowel needs to be passed. This can be acutely uncomfortable for the patient, and the presence of the nurse will do much to alleviate their anxieties and lessen the trauma of the procedure. Recurrent volvulus and intussusception may require surgery (sigmoid resection).

Acute diverticulitis

Diverticula are outpouches of the submucous and mucous layers of the intestine bulging out through the muscle wall of the colon, usually occurring in the sigmoid colon. Diverticulitis arises when the pouches become inflamed.

Incidence. This is a common condition in elderly people in the Western world thought to be due to the low fibre content of their diet.

Causes. It is believed to be a result of changes in bowel motility and increased pressure within the colon due to lack of bulk in the faeces.

Symptoms. Diverticula are often symptomless. Complications may be avoided by introducing a high-fibre diet (see chapter 2).

Distinguishing features

The patient experiences pain, which is usually sudden and severe, initially in the left iliac fossa. It is often described as constant, but may spread across to the whole lower abdomen and is exacerbated by movement. On examination, a palpable tender mass may be detected in the left iliac fossa. There may be rebound tenderness and left-sided pain on pressure to the right side of the abdomen.

Distension, flatulence and belching is often experienced when the pain begins. This is believed to be due to 'mild colonic obstruction caused by the smooth muscle hypertrophy of the bowel wall' (Browse 1984).

On questioning the patient will probably have previously experienced altered bowel habits alternating between constipation and diarrhoea. This is because most symptoms attributed to uncomplicated diverticula are due to inflammatory bowel disease.

Pyrexia, tachycardia, malaise and progressive weakness are also seen in acute diverticulitis.

Diverticulitis is treated with antibiotics, and patients who are severely ill with pain, pyrexia and tachycardia may well be starved for a few days in order to rest the gut. There is some debate as to whether or not longer-term management should include a high-fibre intake. On the one hand, a high-fibre intake stimulates peristalsis and movement of faeces through the gut, while on the other hand, it is thought that fibre bulk may exacerbate the condition in some patients. Generally, it is advisable that patients should eat foods which they can digest easily, drink as much fluid as they can (preferably 2 L/day), and take regular exercise to encourage colonic peristalsis.

In an acute phase, the inflamed colon and peritoneum may adhere to other structures. The eroding infection may then cause a fistula, e.g. into the bladder or vagina which would allow faecal contents to enter them. The patient may complain of passing flatus through the urethra or vagina, with faecal contamination of urine or vaginal secretions. Fistulae are treated by defunctioning the gut. A temporary stoma is formed, allowing healing of the fistula (see Ch. 4 for stomatherapy).

CONCLUSION

The acute abdomen has many possible origins and causes, as outlined above. The treatment and care are underpinned by the experience, skill and knowledge of the nurses. Prompt action based on intelligent rationale is crucial to saving life and minimising complications, while sensitivity, awareness and shrewdness are paramount in supporting and advising, not only sufferers, but also friends and families.

The acute phase often brings with it implications for changes in lifestyle. This may be for a period of months or it may be for the foreseeable future. In some cases, these changes, if not effected, can lead to recurrence, if not death (e.g. alcohol consumption and pancreatitis). Therefore, support from social peers and family in these changes is essential following discharge. This is often best obtained by involving them, along with the patient, in the process of education about the disease and prevention of its recurrence. The nurse is the lynchpin in the success of this education. With sound experience and knowledge, not only of the clinical aspect of caring for someone with such a condition, but also of the basis of successful health promotion, successful outcomes of care will be achieved.

REFERENCES

Alfaro R 1990 Applying nursing diagnosis and the nursing process, 2nd edn. Lippincott, Philadelphia

Bailey R, Clarke M 1991 Stress and coping in nursing. Chapman & Hall, London

Bond M K, Pearson I 1969 Psychological aspects of pain in women with cancer of the cervix. Psychosomatic Research 13:13–19

Browse N 1984 An introduction to the symptoms and signs of surgical disease. Edward Arnold, London, Ch 16

Forrest A, Carter D, MacLeod I 1991 Principles and practice of surgery. Churchill Livingstone, Edinburgh

Gibson H B (ed.) 1994 Psychology of pain and anaesthesia. Chapman and Hall, London

Griffiths D 1980 Psychological and social aspects of pain. Nursing 1:1–7

Hayward J 1975 Information, a prescription against pain. RCN London

Kumar P J, Clark M L 1994 Clinical medicine, 3rd edn. Baillière Tindall, London

McCaffery M 1972 Nursing management of the patient with pain. J B Lippincott Company, Philadelphia.

Mobily P, Herr K, Kelley L 1993 Cognitive behavioural techniques to reduce pain; a validation study. International Journal Nursing Standard 30(6):537–548

FURTHER READING

Burkitt H G, Quick C, Gatt D 1996 Essential surgery, problems, diagnosis and management. Churchill Livingstone, Edinburgh

Jackson A 1995 Acute pain: its physiology and the pharmacology of analgesia. Nursing Times 91(16):27–28

McLance K, Heuther S (eds) 1994 Patho-physiology – The biological basis for disease in adults and children, 2nd edn. Mosby St Louis, Ch 7

Melzack R, Wall P D 1988 Challenge of Pain. Penguin, London

Malignancies of the gastrointestinal tract

Teresa Finlay

INTRODUCTION

As more than 25% of cancers diagnosed in England and Wales (OPCS 1992) are primary tumours of the gastrointestinal (GI) tract, it is not surprising that most nurses caring for adult patients in any clinical setting will encounter people with a malignancy of the GI tract at some time. A background of factual knowledge, in addition to an understanding of the emotional issues involved, helps nurses to develop and deliver nursing care appropriately. Medical practitioners often express pessimism and feelings of failure about their experiences of treating patients with digestive tract malignancy, which inevitably colours the impressions of those working with them. Nurses in specialist gastroenterology or oncology units (clinics, endoscopy suites or wards) will meet these patients more frequently and will have had opportunities to consider their own feelings about caring for patients with these malignancies. It is important for practitioners to have considered what their own concerns and anxieties would be, were they to find themselves in the patients' situation, however frequently such patients are encountered. Awareness of one's own feelings, which are integral to the caring approach to patients, whether obvious or not, enables sensitive and objective care.

Assessment is a major part of nursing and is a constant and evolving process. Frameworks in the form of nursing models give structure to assessment, and the author had chosen to use Roy's (1976) model as a framework for considering more commonly occurring GI tract malignancies. (This is not intended to be prescriptive, as each nurse will choose their own framework.) Roy (1976) identified four modes of behaviour: physiological, self-concept, interdependence and role function. Consideration will be given to how people diagnosed with a carcinoma of the digestive tract may adapt to their altered state in each of the modes in turn, and how nursing intervention can facilitate their adaptation. In considering the physiological aspects of a patient's adaptation to digestive tract cancers, malignancies of specific anatomical areas will be examined separately in some detail. The impact of a diagnosis of cancer on the other three modes of behaviour will be considered with a more generalised overview, as experiences are not necessarily distinctly related to the cancer diagnosed – specific information is given where appropriate. Whilst this will provide useful generalised information, it is worth remembering that since no patients, cancers or nurses are the same, both nurses and patients will draw on numerous resources for knowledge and will apply this to their own unique experiences of disease or of caring for patients and their families.

PHYSIOLOGICAL MODE

In this area of assessment, nurses focus on the physical effects of a disease on an individual patient, but a broader knowledge of the scientific or empirical basis of the problem is necessary to enhance nursing skills. This section will address the histology, epidemiology and aetiological factors involved in the more commonly occurring digestive tract cancers in England and Wales (the author is limited by OPCS figures from England and Wales, rather than deliberately wishing to exclude other parts of the world). In the more commonly occurring digestive tract cancers, the varying incidence in different populations in the world (epidemiology) indicate that there are significant environmental factors involved. Furthermore the association of incidence with increasing age would indicate that the environmental effects are cumulative. This provides some clue to their aetiology. As the GI tract is often described as an 'external' organ exposed to the environment, it is reasonable to conclude that it is exposure to different foods/environments during one's lifetime which contribute to the development of some malignant growths in the digestive tract. The importance of staging tumours, possible treatment options, genetic factors and the debate about screening will be discussed. (It is assumed by the author that the digestive tract commences at the oesophagus, and so tumours of the oropharynx are not discussed. Similarly, as primary cancers of the liver are rare in the UK, neither these, nor hepatology generally, will be discussed in this book.)

The oesophagus

Table 7.1 shows that oesophageal cancers are not particularly common in the population, but incidence is increasing more rapidly than any other tumour in the West – by 7%/year. More alarmingly, oesophageal cancer patients have a very poor survival to 5 years. This is principally due to the tumours' rapid growth, early invasion and late diagnosis. As incidence rises with age, particularly in women, anorexia and weight loss may well be assumed to be part of the process of ageing by patient, family and General Practitioner (GP) alike. Other symptoms of heartburn and indigestion are not uncommon throughout life and are also often ignored for considerable lengths of time. Indeed, development of Barrett's oesophagus – columnar lined oesophagus with small intestinal metaplasia proximal to the OGJ – arises as a result of chronic reflux of acidic gastric contents and is thought to predispose some patients to developing a carcinoma (Kumar et al 1992). But the onset of dysphagia (the most common presenting symptom) indicates obstruction of 50% of the

Table 7.1 Summary of the epidemiology, aetiology and histology of GI tract cancers (collated with information from OPCS 1992)

Anatomical area	Incidence [Figures only for England and Wales (OPCS 1992)]	Male/female ratio	Death rate	Survival rate	Epidemiology	Aetiological factors	Principal histological type
Oesophagus	Increases with age, peaking for men at 65–69, for women at 75–79 years. Upward trend in E & W	3:2	1:5000 per year	30% to a year <8% to 5 years	Variable incidence worldwide. Linked to Asian ethnicity, particularly the Chinese	Alcohol consumption, smoking in more affluent populations, malnutrition in less affluent	Upper two-thirds of oesophagus: 95% squamous cell carcinoma Gastro-oesophageal junction: principally adenocarcinoma – much less common
Stomach	Increases with age. Until recently most common occurring cancer worldwide, now second to lung cancer. Decreasing trend worldwide	3:2	1:3000	10% to 5 years	Incidence highest in Japan and east Asia	Association with salted, cured foods, alcohol and a lack of fresh fruit and vegetables and vitamin C Possibly associated with *Helicobacter pylori*	Predominantly adenocarcinoma, subdivided into intestinal and diffuse types Occasionally lymphoma
Biliary tree	Rare	2:3	1:67 000	20% to 5 years	Seen in east-Asian populations due to infestation with liver flukes	Associated with biliary stasis	Adenocarcinoma (cholangio-carcinoma)

Table 7.1 (cont'd)

Anatomical area	Incidence [Figures only for England and Wales (OPCS 1992)]	Male/female ratio	Death rate	Survival rate	Epidemiology	Aetiological factors	Principal histological type
Pancreas	Incidence increases with age, peaking at 70–80 years. Doubled in the last 40 years	1:1	1:5000	10% to a year Unlikely to 5 years	Distribution similar worldwide	Only common factor seems to be smoking	Commonly ductal adenocarcinoma
Ileum	Extremely rare	1:1	1:180 000	Insufficient data	Insufficient data	Possibly Crohn's disease	Lymphoma and carcinoid
Colon and rectum	Increases exponentially with age	3:2	1:500	35–40% to 5 years	Increases with affluent Western populations; low in developing countries	Related to low-fibre, high-fat diet and lack of physical exercise. Major genetic influence in some cases	95% adenocarcinoma
Anus	Extremely rare	3:4	1:270 000	Insufficient data	Insufficient data	Possible association with pre-existing benign condition and AIDS	Squamous cell carcinoma

lumen of the oesophagus by the tumour. Weight loss is then dramatic, particularly as dysphagia progresses from solid foods to soft foods and then to liquids. Some patients ignore symptoms to the point where they first present in an advanced state of malnutrition, dehydration and possibly with aspiration pneumonia due to 'overspill' of food and saliva into the trachea and bronchi.

Diagnostic investigations include

- barium studies (give information as to tumour site and length, peristalsis, and organ displacement; contours of the tumour margins indicate difference between benign and malignant lesions)
- oesophago-gastroscopy (biopsies can be taken and histology ascertained)
- chest X-rays
- computed tomography (CT) scanning to assess operability
- liver ultrasound scan for metastases.

Staging, as with any malignancy, is vital in order to inform decision-making by both patient and clinicians as to the appropriate courses of treatment or palliation. In oesophageal cancer, a tumour, node, metastasis (TNM) classification as proposed by the Union Internationale Contre le Cancer (UICC), or modification thereof, is commonly used to stage tumours. TNM classifications stage a malignancy in three parts:

T – primary tumour
N – lymph node involvement
M – distant metastases.

On diagnosis, fewer than 10% of patients are likely to have curable tumours, treatment of which finds them alive 5 years later.

Treatment of some kind is almost always suitable for patients with oesophageal cancer, in order to relieve their distressing symptoms and improve quality of life for some time. When a cure is considered possible, radical resection of the tumour is required. Reconstruction of the oesophagus is then performed, either by mobilising the stomach and moving it up into the thoracic cavity, or by transposing a section of colon into the thorax connecting the resection margins. (Details of surgery cannot be given here; the reader is referred to relevant texts cited at the end of the chapter.) However, patients undergoing resection, whether aimed at cure or palliation, will require considerable pre-operative preparation in terms of the following:

- protein, calorie and vitamin intake prior to surgery to maximise healing, homeostasis and immune system function
- what surgery involves immediately
- how they can be directly involved in planning their care
- what to expect as regards pain and its control
- respiratory support (a thoracic (incision) approach is often used) and postoperative physiotherapy (this may require a period of ventilation and a stay in a high-dependency unit (HDU) depending on the hospital facilities)

- complete starvation for a period of several days postoperatively to facilitate anastomotic healing
- the use of several infusion and drainage tubes including a chest drain and a nasogastric tube (these may be required for several days to reduce pressure on, and facilitate healing of, the anastomosis – patients experience significant irritation from them)
- having considerably altered eating patterns for life postoperatively – the capacity of the stomach is likely to be much reduced depending on the altered anatomy of the upper GI tract after resection
- collaboration with dieticians is vital in order to plan and implement a new nutritional regime which will provide sufficient nutrients and fluid with the upper GI tract's altered capacity, taking into account the patient's food preferences
- preparation of the patient and family for the possibility of an inoperable tumour.

Oseophageal resection is a dangerous surgical procedure. The potential for usual surgical complications is increased by the severe pain these patients can experience postoperatively. Their ability to maintain adequate respiratory function and alveolar expansion, or to move effectively to stimulate peripheral circulation, is significantly reduced. Sepsis and anastomotic leak or breakdown can be fatal. Most importantly for nurses, it should be emphasised that this is a frightening experience for patients who need the continuity and moral support, as well as clinical expertise, of nurses whom they know and have come to trust.

Where there is nursing expertise and adequate staffing resource to support it, it is the author's experience that patients undergoing oesophageal resection will recover more quickly with fewer complications if nursed continuously in the surgical ward to which they were initially admitted. A period in a separate HDU is disruptive and frightening for patients, even if pre-operative visits are possible. The lack of continuity of nursing by familiar staff is not conducive to recovery. However, it must be stressed that nursing expertise – particularly in managing and titrating analgesia – in epidural or intravenous patient-controlled analgesia (PCA) infusions, medical staff availability over a 24-h period and sufficient resourcing are required to enable this approach to care.

Other treatment approaches include radiotherapy. This may be used radically for tumours of the upper third of the oesophagus; pre-operatively to shrink tumours and facilitate resection; post-operatively; or as a palliative treatment. Radiotherapy of the upper GI tract is likely to induce nausea and vomiting. In large doses there may be pulmonary fibrosis or possible spinal cord damage. The initial mucosal reaction is likely to exacerbate dysphagia, and mucositis persists for some weeks. There is a high risk of broncho-oesophageal fistula development in these patients.

Chemotherapy has previously been of limited value. The side-effects of nausea, vomiting, stomatitis and diarrhoea add insult to injury for patients who are already considerably debilitated. However, as some oesophageal tumours are chemosensitive and drug trials are being conducted, this treatment option (usually in combination with radiotherapy) is being pursued by some as a realistic alternative to risk-associated surgery.

The principal treatment aims are palliative, with symptomatic relief of dysphagia and pain control being the prime concerns. As the oesophageal cancer progresses, pain, malnutrition and cachexia, and dehydration become the patient's main problems. Dilatation of the oesophagus may be repeated several times via an endoscope. Rigid oesophageal tubes (such as the Celestin tube) may also be inserted to maintain the lumen and can provide relief of dysphagia for some time. Self-expanding metal stents can be placed in the lumen of the oesophagus via an endoscope. These metallic stents are advantageous because, being small, they are easy to insert through tight tumour strictures. Once they are in position, they gradually expand to dilate the malignant strictures with minimal trauma, also achieving symptom relief for some time. Alternatively, the use of laser therapy (performed under sedation via endoscope) ablates the tumour, may be repeated and provides relief of symptoms, although it does not prevent spread of the tumour to surrounding and distant organs. Risks associated with this treatment are perforation of the oesophagus or haemorrhage; patients who are reaching the later stages of the disease may not survive subsequent treatments. Patients experience retrosternal pain after laser therapy, dilatation and tube insertion, and should be warned to expect this, although it can be relieved by medication. Eating and drinking may be recommenced after recovery from the sedation. The position of a Celestin tube may need to be checked with a chest X-ray, and patients require information and education about eating soft foods and drinking carbonated drinks after meals in order to maintain the patency of the tube.

In the opinion of some clinicians, it is a priority to maintain nutritional intake, and some patients may be offered gastrostomy feeding to maintain nutrition and hydration while total dysphagia is developing. The ethics of such an intervention may be questioned. Arguably, gastrostomy feeding prolongs life, as well as the cancer's life, but what quality of life can be achieved for the individual? Alternatively, the opposite situation can arise where a patient wishes to have every available moment of life, regardless of the potentially poor quality of that time. Nurses may find themselves involved in uncomfortable dilemmas relating to such decisions for ongoing supportive therapy. They need to keep themselves informed of the patient's understanding of the situation, and their needs and desires in this matter, in order to represent them.

The stomach

Carcinoma of the stomach used to be one of the most common malignancies in the developed world, but its incidence is now declining worldwide. However, this provides little hope for the person diagnosed with a cancer of the stomach, as, despite improvements in anaesthesia, surgery and nursing care, only 10% of patients treated are alive after 5 years.

As with oesophageal tumours, the symptoms patients experience do not differ initially from usual experiences of indigestion or 'upset stomach', and herein lies the problem. People may well already be used to chronic indigestion, for example, and will not seek medical advice for symptoms they have self-diagnosed and treated with over-the-counter preparations for some time. As time progresses, symptoms may include feeling distended and particularly full after eating. Weight loss will occur, possibly with nausea and vomiting, weakness and anaemia (due to small haemorrhages from the friable tumour tissue into the stomach). Retrosternal or back pain may be experienced, and darkened stool or malaena may be noticed if there has been a significant bleed. Unfortunately, the symptoms which provoke consultation with a doctor usually only occur at a reasonably advanced stage of the disease. When there is pyloric obstruction due to tumour growth, patients will experience dramatic weight loss and dehydration. They will vomit undigested food regularly and in small amounts as 'overflow' occurs on top of chronic distension. In tumours involving the fundus or cardia, patients may have some dysphagia accompanying other symptoms. It is interesting to note that adenocarcinomas in the lower third of the oesophagus are thought to arise in the stomach at the cardia, and to spread up into the oesophagus under the mucosa, only becoming superficially evident in the oesophagus (Kumar et al 1992) – hence the similarities in surgery for patients with middle and lower third oesophageal tumours and tumours of the fundus or cardia.

In physiological assessment, experienced nurses will ascertain specifically:

- whether the patient has a prior history of dyspepsia, and what, if any, medications the patient has taken previously in an attempt to treat their symptoms. (These may initially be as effective in alleviating symptoms from a carcinoma as those from benign ulceration.) Duration of symptoms is important, particularly the time over which weight loss has occurred and to what degree.
- current dietary and eating habits (recent changes and over what period). These are important in planning the nourishment to be arranged for the patient both initially and in the future. Again, it is likely to be appropriate to involve a dietician at the earliest stage, regardless of future treatment plans, in order to maximise available nutritional resources for the patient;
- other symptoms associated with the gut and eating, such as distension and fullness, increased eructation, nausea, indigestion, or reflux.
- any reports of vomiting, which should prompt enquiry into associations with eating and an assessment of its appearance, whether coffee-ground or streaked with fresh blood.
- the patient's bowel habit, and any alterations in frequency or colour of faeces. Haemorrhage may be visible or occult and both can cause the patient to become anaemic; contributing to weakness and lethargy. Presence of blood in the faeces is an irritant to the colon and may cause loose stool or diarrhoea.
- pain; whether it is associated with eating, an empty stomach or any other activities, and also any medication used to alleviate it, and the effectiveness of this medication.

- the patient's general appearance and colour, which may provide indications of anaemia and cachexia.

Investigations to achieve diagnosis include the following:

- gastroscopy enables visualisation of the ulcer and samples will be taken for histological examination; both tissue biopsies and brushings of the cells of the mucosa will be taken for analysis
- barium double-contrast studies of the stomach (coating the gastric mucosa with barium and then introducing air) define the mucosa and show filling defects as well as mucosal irregularities, indicating benign or malignant ulceration
- CT or magnetic resonance imaging (MRI) scans may be used to ascertain the extent of tumour infiltration and spread in assessing suitability for resection
- ultrasound is used principally to scan the liver for metastases.

As with oesophageal cancer, staging of the extent and spread of the tumour will indicate the prognosis, and viable treatment options may then be chosen. Staging is classified using a TNM classification similar to that explained earlier, but again patients often present with symptoms only when the cancer is too advanced to expect realistically to cure it (see Table 7.1). Unless the patient is in an advanced stage of disease and severely debilitated, surgery is the first choice of intervention for symptom relief, and is the only one with any hope of achieving a cure. Radiotherapy and/or chemotherapy may be indicated with or without surgery, although their role in the control of this cancer is felt by some to be limited (Burkitt et al 1996). Decisions about which mode of treatment is appropriate depend on the location of the tumour within the stomach, its stage, the age and general nutritional state of the patient and their choice of suitable options available.

As is the case for patients being prepared for oesophageal resection, those expecting to undergo surgical treatment will require detailed explanation and discussion about the surgery, its expected effects, their role in care planning and their participation, such as deep breathing and leg exercises. Where a thoracic approach is anticipated, the same conditions will apply as those described for oesophageal resection. Regardless of surgical approach, all patients require nutritional support preoperatively, as cancer cachexia and weight loss will have disrupted a healthy nutritional state. Depletion of fat stores and muscle mass will require protein, calorie and vitamin A and C supplementation to maximise healing and immunity.

Patients expecting to have partial or total resection of the stomach will require detailed and repeated discussion regarding future nutritional needs and how to meet them with small, frequent, high-protein meals.

In addition, patients who have had partial or total gastrectomy, whether for oesophageal or gastric carcinoma, need to be warned about dumping syndrome and postprandial hypoglycaemia. Dumping syndrome occurs soon after eating and appears to be related to early emptying of the stomach into the duodenum. A high level of carbohydrate exerts osmotic pressure on the duodenal mucosa, drawing water into the lumen of the gut. This results in nausea, tachycardia, increased blood pressure, sweating, weakness and feeling faint. Diarrhoea may occur and some improvement can be felt after vomiting. Postprandial hypoglycaemia has similar effects to dumping syndrome, though less severe, but occurs for different reasons, up to 3 hours after eating. Because the upper GI tract has been shortened, food arrives in the ileum much more quickly than usual. Carbohydrate is rapidly absorbed and results in insulin secretion from the pancreas, causing a reactive hypoglycaemia with similar symptoms to those described above.

Once these conditions have been described to them, patients should be advised to plan their meals as follows (Bibbings 1991):

• high protein intake
• reduced sugar and salt intake
• reduced carbohydrate intake, avoiding high carbohydrate foods
• take fluids between meals as opposed to with food
• take small meals five or more times a day
• rest after meals.

Patients who have radical or total gastrectomy will require vitamin B_{12} supplementation (hydroxycobalamin injections) at 3-monthly intervals to avoid megaloblastic anaemia, and will require explanations of the condition and of the need for supplementation.

Patients also need to be prepared for, and supported in the eventuality of, planned surgery being impossible and either a palliative bypass operation being performed (refer to recommended surgical text Burkitt et al 1996) or no surgical intervention being feasible at all.

Screening for this cancer is being found to be effective in reducing mortality in Japan where the incidence of gastric carcinoma is the highest in the world. Tools used include double-contrast radiology, endoscopy or analysis of gastric secretions. However, in view of the lower incidence in the UK, it is not feasible to screen the population generally. People who have pernicious anaemia or who have had previous gastric surgery are thought to be particularly at risk and may be offered screening.

The biliary tree

Cancers of the biliary tree are usually adenocarcinomas and are otherwise referred to as cholangiocarcinoma. They are comparatively rare in the UK, and a perceived increase in occurrence is more likely to be related to improved diagnostic procedures than a true increase in incidence. Untreated, those diagnosed with a cholangiocarcinoma will probably die within a year; the tumour is characterised by local spread and deep invasion of surrounding structures. It directly spreads to the liver and patients may suffer cholangitis. The combination of cholangitis and local invasion results in death.

Patients first tend to be aware of any problem when obstructive jaundice develops. If the tumour arises in the upper third of the biliary tree (above the cystic duct and junction of the right and left hepatic ducts) and the patient is jaundiced, then the growth is well established and has infiltrated the duct to a point below the merging of right and left ducts. Tumours in the remainder of the bile duct will give rise to symptoms of jaundice earlier. However, pain is less likely to be a problem for these patients, unless they have gallstones. Biliary calculi are associated with tumours arising in the gall bladder itself. In advanced tumours, the patient may have a firm, enlarged liver and ascites, portal hypertension and the symptoms of liver failure.

This disease commonly affects people between the ages of 50 and 70 years, and by the time jaundice develops the tumour is usually well established. A physiological nursing assessment will focus on the following points:

- when did the patient first notice symptoms that caused concern and what were they?
- if/when was any fever of unknown origin noticed?
- when was jaundice first noticed?
- any alteration in dietary habit; likes and dislikes
- weight loss – how much and over what period?
- any pain, its intensity, when it occurs and what relieves it
- altered appearance of urine – is bilirubin present?
- altered bowel habit and colour of stools – steatorrhoea?
- other symptoms associated with jaundice, pruritus – what does the patient usually do to relieve it?

Patients may well associate their symptoms with a benign condition such as gallstones or hepatitis – although this may be just as frightening – and may not anticipate a diagnosis of malignancy. This is not surprising, as this cancer is rare in incidence among most patients' circles of friends and family. During the process of investigation and diagnosis, as with any patient, nurses can provide support and consolation with a sensitive presence. It may be suitable for an experienced nurse to discuss with some patients the possible findings of the battery of tests they are subjected to. Whilst it is not suitable to speculate about definitive results, in certain circumstances giving a patient the opportunity to consider potential findings may allay unecessary fears or give more time for bad news to be confronted.

Cholangiocarcinoma is commonly diagnosed with ultrasound (potentially including ultrasound-guided fine-needle aspiration), possibly CT scanning, and most commonly by cholangiography (ERCP).

In the UK, there is no nationally accepted staging framework for biliary cancers, and treatment approaches vary according to the extent of involvement of the ducts, the liver and surrounding structures such as the inferior vena cava, and whether there are distant metastases. Potential treatment includes intubation of the obstructed bile duct by a stent draining into the duodenum. Radiotherapy and resection – whether aimed at cure or palliation – have a limited role. Chemotherapy also has limited use in treating cholangiocarcinoma. Palliative intubation of the duct through the tumour is the mainstay of treatment and will relieve the jaundice, its associated symptoms and cholangitis. However, stents do not remain patent reliably, resulting in recurrent obstructive symptoms and cholangitis, and require replacement periodically.

Preparing patients for surgical treatment may include preparing them for the likely possibility of the procedure proving palliative. Even those patients thought to have had a curative operation usually succumb to recurrent disease and invasion of surrounding structures, including the liver and major vessels. Resection of the tumour, surrounding lengths of duct, lymphatics and possibly the liver also require major reconstructive procedures and considerable pre-operative preparation and aftercare similar to that for pancreatectomy.

Pancreas

The mention of pancreatic cancer usually provokes a feeling of gloom in most clinical practitioners familiar with it. This is not surprising as the likelihood of surviving pancreatic cancer for 5 years is less than 1%. Tumours of the pancreas are commonly ductal adenocarcinoma and may arise in the head, the body or the tail of the pancreas. For aetiological purposes, it is interesting to note that the incidence of this cancer has been rising in the last 40 years, although the short prognosis for those diagnosed precludes further research into possible causes (OPCS 1992).

Growths in the head of the gland are usually smaller and diagnosed somewhat earlier than those in the body or the tail, as symptoms are evident earlier with closer proximity to the gut and common bile duct. Sadly, though, it is obstructive jaundice which is the most common presenting sign of cancers of the head of the pancreas, and if the tumour has obstructed the common bile duct or the ampulla of Vater, it is unlikely that the patient will survive more than a year from diagnosis. Jaundice will be accompanied by pruritus, dark urine and light-coloured stools. The other two main symptoms are pain and colossal weight loss – up to 15 kg in a few weeks.

The pain experienced by people with cancer of the head of pancreas may be distinctive. Initially it may be confused with indigestion and gaseous distension, but becomes more severe, possibly radiating from the epigastric region to the right upper quadrant or through to the patient's back. It is likely to be affected by posture, activity and eating, and is relieved by lying flat or sitting, leaning forwards.

Weight loss is dramatic because of reduced digestive enzyme secretion and consequent malabsorption, and reduced insulin production resulting in hyperglycaemia.

Tumours arising in the body of the pancreas are associated with severe epigastric pain, often occurring several hours after eating, and often with vomiting. It may be relieved by lying in a foetal position or sitting forwards. Whilst not continuous in nature, this experience is reported by some patients as extremely frightening and associated with imminent death. Cancers in the tail of the pancreas are often first diagnosed by finding metastases; spread is initially to localised lymph nodes and structures, including the duodenum, bile duct, spleen, colon, portal and splenic veins, and peritoneal cavity, and later to the liver and lungs. Pain occurs in the upper abdomen, radiating to the left hypochondrium, and is not as intense as that experienced with cancer of the head or body of the pancreas. Patients with cancers in the body or tail are unlikely to become jaundiced and have more vague symptoms of weakness and lethargy, weight loss and anorexia.

As with other upper GI tract cancers, ultrasonography and CT scanning may be used initially. Ultrasound scanning shows masses, dilated bile ducts and liver metastases, while CT gives more exact tumour extent and location. In carcinoma of the head of the pancreas, ERCP is usually conducted to demonstrate the obstruction of the ampulla, to obtain tissue samples for histology, and possibly to 'stent' the tumour through the ampulla and common bile duct and provide relief of the obstructive jaundice. As with aforementioned tumours, pancreatic cancers in particular are associated with late 'onset' of symptoms and diagnosis at too late a stage to even consider attempts at curative procedures.

On initial meeting with nurses, patients may or may not have an inkling of what is wrong with them. It is particularly difficult for many nurses to reconcile their own feelings with these situations, as the prognosis is so likely to be poor and the patient may have very little time to adapt their behaviour to accept dying within months. However, these patients and their families require nursing care and support as any others. An assessment of their physiological state is not only necessary, it often provides a less emotionally fraught arena from which to start developing a relationship. This provides the basis for broaching the more difficult aspects of assessing their understanding and enabling adaptation to a cancer diagnosis with little hope for the future.

Specific aspects of altered physiology to be aware of in these patients include the following:

- what is the most significant physical symptom or physical change the patient has felt?
- a detailed assessment of pain and what, if anything, relieves it
- is there any jaundice; how long has the patient or their family noticed it; is there pruritus, are there scratch marks; what helps; what is the general condition of the skin?
- what weight loss has occurred and over what time period (this is likely to be significant and frightening to the patient; it is not helpful to them to see shock demonstrated on hearing the response)?
- how have their eating habits changed; what do they eat and drink now; likes and dislikes?
- is there any vomiting; does it have a pattern?
- is urine dark in colour?
- has the patient noticed altered bowel habit, including constipation, diarrhoea, pale or offensive stools which float?
- is there any distension and abdominal discomfort?
- how have the symptoms affected their ability to conduct a usual daily routine, and sleep?

If resection for cancers in the head of the pancreas is to be attempted, a detailed process of preparation is required (as with any major surgery) so that all involved parties (patient and family, surgical team, nurses, physiotherapists, dieticians and pharmacists) are fully aware of the intended procedure, the patient's current state of health and the expected outcome. Resection procedures include total pancreatectomy or Whipple's procedure, where the tail of the pancreas remains and is anastomosed to the jejunum, as are the common bile duct and the remainder of the stomach, at different points. The stomach is anastomosed to the jejunum distal to the common bile duct and the pancreas to allow the alkaline juices to enter the jejunum before the acidic gastric juices, so decreasing the potential for ulceration at the gastrojejunostomy site. Vagotomy will reduce the potential for ulceration further. Surgery is complicated and the usual risks of general anaesthesia and immobility are exacerbated by several factors:

- the patient's pre-existing condition
- the duration of surgery and anaesthetic
- the extent of surgery
- the possibility of anastomotic breakdown, fistula formation and leaking enzymes, bile or gastric secretions, all of which are highly damaging to tissues not adapted to containing them.

Intensive nursing care is required postoperatively for patients undergoing resection. Problems include:

- respiratory problems associated with pain, fluid imbalance, hypovolaemia and pneumonia
- circulatory problems with hypotension, tachycardia and low central venous pressure due to hypovolaemia or haemorrhage from wounds internally or externally (altered liver function may derange clotting)
- fluid imbalance with low urine output, oedema and pulmonary oedema, leading to hypovolaemia and shock; fluid losses from the gut and shifting of fluid to the interstitial (third) space as a result of reduced circulating protein levels (including hypoalbuminaemia)
- pain
- breakdown of anastomoses or wounds or development of fistulae with leaking of corrosive digestive juices
- sepsis and fever
- severe nutritional deficiencies requiring total parenteral nutrition and infusions of albumin
- deranged blood glucose regulation requiring sliding scales of insulin
- increased potential for thromboembolus with duration of surgery and subsequent inactivity.

An awareness of what to expect will facilitate recovery on the patient's part and allay anxiety for relatives. It is crucial to their recovery that patients' pain is well controlled, to enable deep breathing, movement and sleep, and that they have an understanding of the importance of early mobilisation postoperatively. Both pre-operatively and after the initial recovery period, consideration will be given to adaptation of eating habits to the patient's drastically altered anatomy and physiology. The stomach's capacity will be reduced, and depending on the extent of pancreatic resection, supplements of pancreatic enzymes will be required, as will adaptation to being an insulin-dependent diabetic.

Other therapeutic approaches have limited application to pancreatic cancer. Radiotherapy in effective doses is not possible due to the gland's proximity to radiosensitive structures such as the kidneys and spinal cord. Radiotherapy, chemotherapy and/or surgery may be suggested for more aggressive regimes, though their efficacy is debatable.

Attempts at curative resection for carcinoma of the pancreas are fraught with high mortality rates associated with surgery or finding non-resectable tumours. In many patients with a tumour in the head of the pancreas, if it is possible, intubation of the ampulla and the common bile duct is the most appropriate intervention to relieve jaundice, with supportive continuing care for symptom relief. Controlling pain, achieving realistic nutritional intake and relieving other symptoms, are the major practical challenges in continuing care for this group of patients.

The ileum

It is rare for patients to develop tumours of the ileum, and those who do usually have a carcinoid (slowly progressing growth) or a lymphoma, both of which commonly arise in the appendix. If the patient is not diagnosed by routine histological reporting on appendicectomy, they may present with small bowel obstruction. The treatment is surgical resection and anastomosis of the ileum or formation of an ileostomy. Consequently, the person usually receives the diagnosis as a shock after emergency surgery. Nursing care and support through the emotional adaptation are most important, while the physical care required is straightforward according to the exact surgery performed.

Carcinoid tumours do not respond to radiotherapy or chemotherapy, although chemotherapy is indicated for patients diagnosed with lymphoma. Naturally this will not commence until some weeks after healing of the surgical wounds is complete and will be dependent on the specific histology of the tumour resected.

Colon and rectum

Adenocarcinomas of the colon and rectum have essentially the same pathology and are responsible for 95% of cancers arising in the large bowel (Hermanek 1989). Thus, they are often referred to collectively as colorectal cancers. Colorectal cancer is an increasing problem in the developed world because it is common (affecting 1 in 500 people in England and Wales) and outcomes for patients have not significantly improved in the last 40 years despite increased understanding of the disease or improved treatment approaches (OPCS 1992).

Colorectal cancer is second only to lung cancer in men and breast cancer in women in the UK as a cause of cancer-related death. As its incidence is linked to age, this implies that causation is due to exposure over time of the colorectum to carcinogenic agents within the environment of the bowel, i.e. the products of digestion over a lifetime. Thus, it is logical that incidence in the anatomical areas of the large bowel are highest in the sigmoid colon and rec-

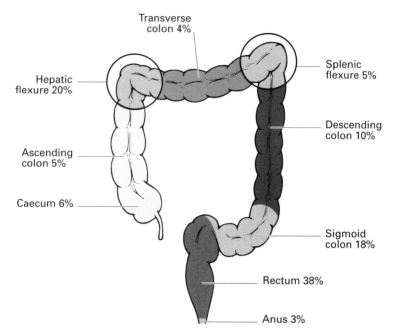

Fig 7.1 Percentage occurrence of colorectal cancer at various sites (after Souhami & Tobias 1995).

tum – where faeces are stored prior to defaecation and have longer contact with the mucosa (see Fig. 7.1). Theories as to aetiology abound, but it is now established that the cancer develops due to the stepwise progressive damage to the genes controlling epithelial cell division and growth. It is less clear what factors cause the DNA to become damaged in those people who do not inherit a genetic abnormality. The most credible theory is based on the association of incidence with a refined, high saturated fat, low-fibre diet (Burkitt 1971, Doll & Peto 1981).

People who have ulcerative colitis (UC) are more liable to develop colorectal cancer, particularly as the interval from diagnosis of UC lengthens (Misiewicz et al 1988). Those with Crohn's colitis are in less danger than UC sufferers but have a higher risk than the unaffected population.

There are also known genetic anomalies associated with colorectal carcinoma. High-risk groups include those with the genes either for familial adenomatous polyposis (FAP), Turcot's syndrome or Gardner's syndrome – where affected individuals inherit a chromosomal abnormality resulting in multiple adenomas in the colon and rectum or throughout the gut. One or more of these polyps will almost certainly become malignant within the first 35 years of life, necessitating removal of the colon and rectum in the case of FAP to avoid death. In Gardner's syndrome, transplant of the entire digestive tract, liver and pancreas has been performed in a few cases with mixed success.

Transplants of the bowel are much more prone to rejection than other organ transplants, although multiple visceral transplants do better than those of the intestine only. However, massive immunosuppression is required which can be self-defeating (Abu-Elmagd et al 1994).

People who inherit 'cancer family' syndromes – called Lynch syndromes – are at risk: those with Lynch I will inherit genetic predisposition to colorectal cancer; those with Lynch II to breast, colorectal, uterine or other adenocarcinoma as well. Most colorectal cancers arise spontaneously, although research is currently being focused on altered DNA coding as a significant contributing factor. Individuals with a first-degree relative (parent or sibling) are known to have an increased risk of developing a cancer themselves, and the younger the person at diagnosis, when there are no other contributing factors, the more likely there is to be a genetic component to their tumour aetiology (see the section on interdependence for problems associated with implications of hereditary illness, p. 185).

Colorectal cancer is thought in most, if not all, cases to be preceded by a benign growth of an adenomatous polyp (as with adenomatous syndromes mentioned above). High-risk groups, which include patients who have already been treated for a colorectal cancer, are currently screened for early cancers with colonoscopy. Given the prevalence of colorectal cancer in this country, it has long been believed by some that a screening programme for the general population would reduce the death rates from the disease. However, certain conditions must apply for a screening programme to be successful, i.e. to significantly reduce the death rate from the disease. These are as follows (Wilson & Jungner 1968):

- The condition screened for must be an important health problem.
- There should be an acceptable treatment for patients with recognised disease.
- Facilities for diagnosis and treatment should be available in sufficient quantity to meet the demands required as a result of screening case-finding.
- The disease should have a recognisable latent or early symptomatic stage.
- The natural course of the disease, including the latent phase to declared disease, should be adequately understood.
- There should be a suitable test or examination.
- This test must be acceptable to the population.
- There should be an agreed policy on whom to treat as patients.
- The cost of case-finding (including diagnosis and treatment of patients) should be economically balanced in relation to possible expenditure on medical care as a whole.
- Case-finding should be a continuing process and not a once-for-all project.

Several problems arise from this. These include firstly that of finding an effective, economically viable but acceptable screening test. It is pointless setting up a screening programme if it has an insufficient detection rate or if the majority of the population are unlikely to comply with the test because they find it distasteful, such as testing one's own faeces for occult blood. Secondly, the financial implications of screening the population, let alone treating them, are enormous and unlikely to be feasible economically within the current health care system in the UK.

Screening depends on finding pre-malignant growths (polyps) or very early cancers in the case of colorectal cancers. There are different staging classifications for colorectal cancers around the world. That commonly encountered in the UK is based on an adaptation of Dukes' classification (Dukes 1930), to which a fourth stage has been added (Fig. 7.2). True staging can only be achieved with surgery and excision of the growth and lymph nodes. Histological examination of the tumour invasion and lymph nodes will define the stage, unless of course there are known liver metastases which indicate a stage D tumour.

Similar to the scenarios described with other GI tract cancers, patients with a colorectal tumour are likely not to be symptomatic for a considerable time after initial invasion of the growth. Symptoms are easily confused with those associated with occasional stomach upsets, or haemorrhoids if there is visible bleeding. Patients may present with altered bowel habit which can mean anything including constipation, loose stool, both of these alternately, abdominal distension, increased flatulence and, if the lesion is in the rectum, feelings of a constantly full rectum and tensemus – feeling the need to evacuate the bowel, but nothing being passed except perhaps mucus which may be blood-stained. Stools may be covered with mucus or fresh blood, or bleeding from the tumour may be occult. There is likely to have been some weight loss and the person may have a degree of anorexia and weakness, particularly if they are anaemic. On investigation, serum levels of the protein carcinoembryonic antigen (CEA) may be raised. This is a tumour marker for colorectal cancer, but is found to be raised in other conditions also and is usually only measured in patients who are being monitored after treatment. People are very unlikely to present early with colorectal cancer unless they are already familiar with the disease. It is embarrassing to discuss one's bowel habit, particularly when one feels symptoms are likely to be transitory and minor. Hence, patients have usually been putting up with discomfort for some time, and depending on the site of the tumour within the colon or rectum, may be diagnosed at an advanced stage of the cancer's growth. If this is the case, they are likely to be anaemic, due to the tumour's occult bleeding, and this is often the symptom that first arouses suspicion, either in the patient or in their doctor. This is particularly frustrating in colorectal cancer, as early detection and treatment are likely to achieve a successful outcome (see Table 7.2).

Patients investigated for colorectal carcinoma are subjected to some of the most degrading and alarming investigations, most of which require the bowel to be clear if they are to be effective. They involve instrumentation of the anus, rectum and colon, whether for colonoscopy, barium enema or rectal ultrasound. All of these tests will elicit the presence and size of a tumour, rectal ultrasound now being used to detect the degree of invasion of the bowel wall by a rectal carcinoma. Liver ultrasound and CT scanning may indicate distant metastases, the liver being the most likely site for secondary tumours

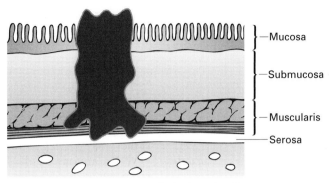

— Mucosa

— Submucosa

— Muscularis

— Serosa

Stage A: localised growth within the bowel wall

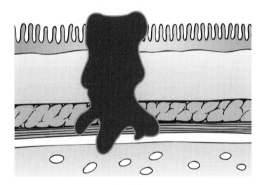

Stage B: growth invaded through the entire thickness of the bowel wall but remains localised

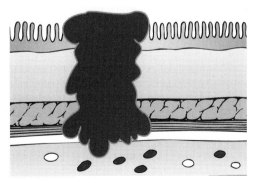

Stage C: invasion through the bowel wall and metastasis to regional lymph nodes

Stage D: tumour with distant metastasis (not shown)

Fig 7.2 Dukes' classification of rectal carcinoma, modified to include a fourth stage (after Dukes 1930).

Table 7.2 Estimated colorectal cancer survival by stage (adapted from Chapuis et al 1987)

Stage at resection	% Survival @ 5 years
Stage A	63–84%
Stage B	51–62%
Stage C	32–44%
Stage D	< 20%

once the lymph nodes are involved. These facts will influence treatment decisions, although the main approach to this cancer is surgery, for either cure or palliation. But, more importantly, the patient often places great faith in these tests despite the indignity of the preparation and most of the tests themselves, inevitably hoping that they will give reason for optimism.

When assessing patients physiologically, the following points will be of particular importance:

- has the patient noticed being more tired and lethargic, and if so, for how long?
- are they anaemic?
- has there been weight loss, and if so, how much and over what period?
- has the patient's diet altered recently; what do they eat habitually; what are any changes in response to?
- how has bowel habit changed; have changes in the appearance of faeces been noticed?
- is there any abdominal distension or visible abdominal mass?
- is there any family history of bowel cancer, or does the patient have a history of colitis?

With a few exceptions, surgical resection of the part of the colon or rectum affected by tumour is the main approach to treatment. Even where resection is unlikely to be curative, this is the favoured option as the effects of progressive disease are appalling: intestinal obstruction, perforation, fungating tumours and invasion of surrounding structures including the genitourinary system may result and cause extreme pain, sepsis and symptoms which can be impossible to manage and lead to unneccesarily traumatic death. However, the prospect of surgery is not to be considered lightly, particularly as many patients who undergo it are elderly and have other physiological problems which may complicate recovery.

Resection of colorectal cancers requires preparation of the bowel before surgery, to facilitate the procedure and healing thereafter. Abdominal surgery is painful and the patient is at more risk of postoperative complications as a result. These two factors alone indicate the need for thorough preparation of the patient in terms of what to expect and how they will be supported and helped to deal with their recovery.

Of specific importance is the patients's nutritional state pre-operatively. They are likely to have lost weight as a result of the tumour growth. The administration of bowel purgatives and starvation for recent investigations will be repeated pre-operatively, depleting available energy and potentially disrupting fluid balance. Assessment and goal setting with dieticians are important to maximise nutritional intake pre-operatively and to maintain fluid balance, even if intravenous fluids are the only possible resource. This is especially important as the gut will not absorb much for 24–72 hours after the operation. Details of postoperative care are similar to that for any other abdominal surgery. The tumour and an approximately 5 cm margin of bowel on either side are resected, after the mesenteric vascular and lymphatic supplies to the area have been dissected out and clamped off. There are two important differences from standard postoperative care:

- the patient and their family will anxiously await the surgeon's prognosis, still hoping for an improvement in prognosis
- only postoperatively will it be known whether the resection has necessitated the formation of a stoma.

While a stoma is not universally required in colorectal cancer resection, many patients associate having bowel cancer with colorectal cancer and thus with having a bag. Surgical techniques have improved considerably, so that low anastomosis of the rectum is now possible. Thus a colostomy is usually formed only when the anus must be excised and abdominoperineal resection is done. An ileostomy or colostomy may serve as a temporary measure to facilitate healing of an anastomosis or inflamed bowel, or as a palliative measure where a tumour is unresectable and the stoma is above it in the bowel, diverting the faecal stream (for details on stoma care, see Ch. 4).

Adjuvant chemotherapy and radiotherapy have been used for some time in an effort to improve outcomes for this group of patients, although 5 year survival rates have not changed in the last 40 years. Radiotherapy is useful in reducing tumour bulk and invasion in rectal cancers before surgery is carried out. It may also reduce spread or recurrence postoperatively in rectal tumours. It is particularly helpful in palliation for inoperable rectal cancers. Irradiating colonic tumours is more difficult as the ileum is radiosensitive at low doses. 5-fluourouracil (5-FU) has been the mainstay of chemotherapy for colorectal cancer, although trials of combinations with other agents are currently underway as adjuncts to surgery.

Early tumours of the rectum (polyps and stage A cancers) may also be resected by trans-anal endoscopic microsurgery (TEM). Via a large endoscope, the entire tumour is excised from the rectal wall without resecting a length of the gut itself. The procedure is much less debilitating for the patient, requiring a hospital stay of only a few days, and avoids the need for a stoma in low cancers. Risks are from haemorrhage, perforation and incomplete excision. This approach is currently only performed in a few specialist centres.

Trans-anal resection or laser therapy may be effective for months or years in controlling rectal tumours which are inoperable, or for patients who cannot withstand major abdominal surgery. Both have low associated morbidity, which is particularly helpful for the elderly, frail person provided they have sufficient home support.

Anus

Anal cancers are rare and are commonly squamous cell carcinomas. Treatment is either by local excision with a wide margin of unaffected tissue or by abdominoperineal resection. This depends on whether the tumour is in the anal canal or on the anal margin, the degree of invasion, the patient's age and ability to handle a stoma, and other factors. Radiotherapy can be effective as an adjunct to surgery, as is chemotherapy; both may be used with local excision rather than radical abdominoperineal resection. Side-effects of chemoradiotherapy include nausea, vomiting, anaemia, leucocytopaenia, thrombocytopaenia, stomatitis and radiation-induced proctitis.

ROLE FUNCTION

Given that most people with a cancer of the digestive tract are diagnosed when over 50 years old, their roles in life are likely to be firmly established. The primary role of gender and age is affected in as much as a person's opinion of their age is coloured by their view of how much of their life they envisage they have left. For example, a previously fit, 50-year-old diagnosed with pancreatic cancer is likely to view their life as being unfairly interrupted, whereas an 80-year-old with a colonic cancer is less likely to do so, and indeed may well succumb to other complications of longevity before the cancer defeats them. In addition, the patient may still be seen as a man or a woman by others, but their own self-perception could be compromised by radical surgery and radiotherapy for rectal carcinoma where there is residual impotence, or rectal and vaginal excision with a permanent colostomy.

The secondary roles are those one cannot change. These include those dictated by relationship to others, such as being a parent, grandparent or sibling, or one's physical state. The tertiary role includes one's chosen roles in life, one's place in local society, whether as a lawyer, a housewife or a retired painter and decorator.

When assessing a person's role function, nurses gain valuable information relating to all other aspects of assessment. In patients with a GI tract cancer, the potential for taking on a new role as a 'cancer patient' and adapting to the conflict imposed by the diagnosis is the focus of assessment. Ascertaining this gives scope for improving the support given to the patient, and also to the family in enabling them to adapt and support the patient themselves.

SELF-CONCEPT

It is unnatural to consider psychological aspects of behaviour and adaptation in isolation, as they are inextricably bound up in all aspects of the person. However, doing so facilitates analysis and information pertinent to this area of care.

In considering a patient's concept of self, nurses are seeking to understand what individuals think and feel about themselves as people, their beliefs about life generally and their own in particular, their moral values and thoughts or anxieties about experiencing an unhealthy state, whether it includes pain, the possibility of altered body shape or function, or the threat of death. Two issues arise from this. Firstly, it is impossible to consider such an assessment unless the assessor has an understanding of his or her own 'self' and is reasonably comfortable with exploring extremely personal information with another person. This is particularly relevant in gastrointestinal oncology. The effects on people of any diagnosis of cancer are usually dramatic, causing crisis confrontation by the sufferer with their self-concept and potential death. This is compounded by potentially devastating physical effects of either a tumour or the relevant treatment to cure or palliate it, such as cachexia and dramatic weight loss which accompanies most GI tract cancers. Secondly, the degree to which such an assessment is conducted is most important. Many nurses do not feel comfortable or confident probing a relative stranger's personal beliefs, and it is arguable that unless one is a trained psychoanalyst, one is not in a position to do so. However, the information gained from understanding how a patient is feeling about what is happening is vital when an holistic approach to care is the priority. At this point it is pertinent to remind the reader that nursing assessment does not have a defined beginning or end within the course of getting to know a patient. In assessing someone's self-concept, early, general impressions can be built on by gentle and subtle open questioning at a later time, when both patient and nurse feel more familiar and comfortable with such a discussion. The dilemma for current and future nursing practice presents a paradox. The perception of decreasing amounts of time to spend quietly getting to know a patient is pitted against the imperative of knowing a patient well in order to give care for them together with their loved ones.

Depending at what point in their disease process one first encounters the patient, they may suspect the diagnosis is one of cancer, or be hoping fervently that it is not, whilst being extremely anxious. Some people appear unusually calm and accepting of whatever is told or done to them without having actually confronted their worst fears at all. They simply hope it will all go away. They may feel at some level that if they are obedient they will be rewarded by good news, and thus seem to be unusually compliant. For example, a patient presenting with jaundice who is to be investigated may have convinced themselves and their family that they have gallstones, and may appear relaxed and even jovial, apparently not considering their 7 kg weight loss in the previous month to be significant. Clearly, something more sinister is likely to be causing the symptoms, but denial, fuelled by lack of familiarity with pancreatic or biliary cancers, is maintaining the possibility of keeping the self-concept intact. In this way, they avoid having to consider the question of severe, chronic and probably fatal illness.

Alternatively, they may already know their diagnosis and may be exhibiting a variety of 'coping' behaviours, such as outward grief and sadness or, more rationally perhaps, some anxiety, fear and hope for improvement of the situation.

In dealing with the disease diagnosis and embarking on unfamiliar experiences, people are usually bombarded by their own emotions, whether they are aware of this or not. Cancer remains one of the most feared diseases in the

Western world, principally because it is unpredictable, leaves the sufferer feeling controlled by the disease and is synonymous with death. In addition, ghastly and painful symptoms may be experienced as a result of an offensive, fungating rectal tumour, and compliance with treatment in no way guarantees cure.

A patient's experience of cancer is unique. There are, however, common themes of disruption to life which nurses should be aware of. As previously stated, the majority of patients will have had their symptoms for some time before either presenting them to a doctor or achieving a diagnosis. Thus, many people feel guilt and anger directed at themselves. Inevitably the 'what if' question arises, and while some are sufficiently emotionally equipped to accept the current situation and begin to deal with it, many people find it enormously difficult to do so. They exhibit their feelings in a variety of behavioural ways, such as projected anger to clinical or hospital staff, uncharacteristic intolerance of minor occurrences, and so on. Anger may not be personally associated. Those who have repeatedly pestered a GP suspecting something sinister and are fobbed off only to have their fears confirmed some time later often blame everyone for something and may present a particular problem in terms of cooperation and understanding.

Nurses assessing this group of patients need to give consideration not only to how the patient feels about his diagnosis and prognosis and his subsequent behaviour, but also to the implications of treatment or the disease process for the individual. Ascertaining how a person handles pain is important in the initial stages of treatment in order to prepare them and help them to do so, but is perhaps more important for future reference. More obviously, there is the question of altered body image, its impact on patients and their perception of how others now view them. In gastrointestinal oncology, this can be a major concern for those who require a stoma, develop a fistula or undergo mutilating surgery.

It is, however, worth considering more discrete aspects of altered body image at this point. The gut is an integral part of everyone's life, usually taken for granted. Whilst there may be no outward sign of alteration, patients who experience extensive gut surgery or radiotherapy may never be able to enjoy a large meal again, or drink several pints of beer with their friends. They may suffer severe constipation, or diarrhoea which ties them to the lavatory. They may be unable to eat their usual food and have to rely on a liquidised diet and nutritious supplements. Alternatively, they may resume their usual physiological behaviour patterns after treatment (for example, after colonic resection and anastomosis for colon cancer) and appear 'normal', but they are still living with an altered impression of their body. It is not appropriate to brush such facts aside in caring for patients – these activities are part of them and it is the nurse's role to enable patients to adapt and cope with changes to optimise their quality of life.

All cancer patients enter a diagnostic phase for life. This is particularly related to the chronic nature of a diagnosis of a digestive tract malignancy. Nurses involved have to be mindful of a patient's continuing exposure to changing stressors – initially, the shock of the diagnosis; perhaps then dealing with painful or disfiguring surgery; possibly going on to experience chemotherapy and/or radiotherapy; followed by the distress of the accompanying lethargy, nausea and vomiting.

As the course of these interventions continues, there is the constant fear of recurrence versus hopes of remission to deal with. Crisis intervention is not applicable if patients are to deal with these stressors over time. Whilst denial may provide respite in dealing with the crisis situation on initial diagnosis, continued denial into later stages of the disease will actively inhibit the patient from adapting to the altered roles in their life in the terminal stages of the illness. Understanding a person's self-concept and likely emotional response to some degree will equip the nurse with important information to enable the patient to adapt to gross and permanent changes in their future lives, whether this be obvious physical changes or dealing with confronting a chronic disease and death. A more positive adaptive response from the patient enhances both their own and their family's quality of life.

INTERDEPENDENCE

Patients presenting with a malignancy of the GI tract are usually bewildered and frightened. Having experienced symptoms which may well have been ignored for some time, they now face a new journey in life, fearful of pain and death – the word cancer being associated with mortality. At this time, the patient's relationships with those significant to them become increasingly important. A nurse's care for a patient is linked to support of the patient's family (this word is used in this text to signify whoever is closest to the patient, related or not). Both the patient's and the family's emotions or perceptions of what is happening will influence the situation.

In the early stage of disease, the patient will be shocked and likely to rely heavily on those closest to them for emotional and practical support. As cancers of the digestive tract affect people more as they get older, many people's closest family are elderly and frail themselves, or are perceived by the patient as being young, too busy and independent. Hence, nurses often encounter situations where either the patient is reluctant to involve their family, or families do not feel the patient should be told their diagnosis. This can pose dilemmas for nurses and doctors, and these situations can only be assessed and handled sensitively on an individual basis with the patient placed at the centre of the experience, their needs and view of their situation taking precedence over everyone's opinion.

A diagnosis of cancer alters both the patient's and their family's view of life for ever. In addition to the physical problems associated with the disease and its treatment, and the possibility of early death, cancer carries a social 'label'. Others' perception of the person changes, as does the patient's own self-perception (see 'self-concept', p. 182). The onset of disease will affect the ability to fulfil previous roles and activities, the anticipation of which is just as frightening as the reality. The family will be just as concerned about this aspect of change as the patient, and all involved will deal with the situation differently. This may pose problems where reactions of family members are incompatible. For example, the patient diagnosed with gastric cancer may deny the problem or its implication in foreshortening his life, but his wife may be devastated and emotionally distressed to the point where she is unable to support him through the early stages of diagnosis and treatment. This will affect communication between them and their mutual ability to adapt to the situation. People's emotional responses to cancer are not predictable and it is often the nurses, as those in closest contact with the patient, who experience the most turbulent emotions of all involved. Knowledge and understanding of both their own feelings and possible reasons for altered behaviour will facilitate the nurse's supportive role. The nurse has a considerable potential to diffuse difficult situations and enable communication, as well as adapting to the changes experienced by patient and relatives.

In assessing a patient, nurses will focus on who is significant to them, what relationship they have with this person(s) and their degree of dependence on each other in emotional, social, financial or practical terms. To an extent, assessment is made of both the patient's and the relatives' behaviour and adaptation in respect of the patient's illness.

Where a diagnosis of a digestive tract cancer has been made, the potential of inheritance is anticipated by relatives, and questions relating to this may well arise. The psychological implications of diagnosis of an inherited component to disease is significant for all involved. The patient, as well as having to handle the new diagnosis and its implications, may be feaful for children and grandchildren. They may experience guilt at having handed on such an inheritance. Powerful emotions can be heightened by the inability to change the situation. Coping strategies are important in helping the patient through an emotionally critical time. Similarly, those potentially affected with a genetic predispostion to colon cancer, for example, may experience anger and guilt themselves. Alternatively, a more optimistic view is that they will be more lucky than the patient, being offered screening for early disease and thus being 'protected' from the same fate.

Many people want to know how to avoid getting the cancer their relative or friend has, or how to protect their children. Giving such advice requires an understanding of the aetiology (for which there is still a lack of clear evidence) of these cancers. It should not be based on a nurse's personal opinions or preferences and should be given in addition to a medical specialist's assessment of the patient's individual risk. Care must be taken not to mislead people with unrealistic promises or, alternatively, with goals for health which are impractical and which the person being advised may not wish to achieve anyway. As digestive tract cancers appear to be related to lifetime exposure to carcinogenic agents, it is unlikely that adult patients in middle age will significantly alter outcomes with changed diet. Advice about healthy eating and lifestyle can improve health generally. Points to include in such advice are as follows:

- assess the person's idea of health and negotiate realistic health goals
- consider dietary intake: five portions of fresh fruit or vegetables a day are recommended, in combination with a low fat diet

- alcohol intake should be moderate, with alcohol-free days
- exercise should be taken regularly as tolerated (if the person is unfit, ill or infirm) and excessive stress avoided over the long term
- the patient should be told to give up smoking if at all possible, or at least reduce tobacco use.

Patients with GI tract cancers meet numerous nurses, doctors and other health care personnel in the course of their illness and its treatment. Rather than individual nurses seeing the patient's experience solely in the light of their own encounter with them, it is useful to consider the patient's experience as central, with the issues pertinent to the patient being dealt with by clinicians around them. There are key points within the journey, such as the first appointment with the GP, the diagnosis of a cancer, a decision about treatment, follow-up appointments after treatment is complete, recurrence, continuing care and death. In Fig. 7.3, it can be seen how many different nurses could be involved in the process, and it should be anticipated how confusing all these different people's roles may seem. Although it may seem obvious at one level, communication between practitioners about the patient and their

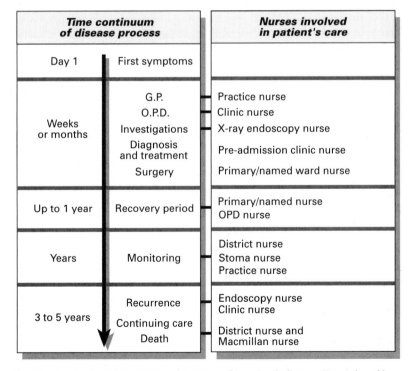

Time continuum of disease process		Nurses involved in patient's care
Day 1	First symptoms	
Weeks or months	G.P.	Practice nurse
	O.P.D.	Clinic nurse
	Investigations	X-ray endoscopy nurse
	Diagnosis and treatment	Pre-admission clinic nurse
	Surgery	Primary/named ward nurse
Up to 1 year	Recovery period	Primary/named nurse OPD nurse
Years	Monitoring	District nurse Stoma nurse Practice nurse
3 to 5 years	Recurrence	Endoscopy nurse Clinic nurse
	Continuing care Death	District nurse and Macmillan nurse

Fig 7.3 Nursing contributions over the course of a patient's disease. (Reproduced by kind permission of Nursing Times where this first appeared in the Professional Development series on 'digestive tract cancers' on December 13 1995.)

treatment is highly important to the patient's perception that their care is meaningful and understood by all involved. As health care becomes more specialised, it is more likely to appear segmented to the receiver, and this can engender anxiety about being forgotten or inappropriately treated at a time when people feel most vulnerable and frightened.

With the number of nurses involved, it would seem logical to reduce and share the perceived workload in terms of nursing assessment. Valuable information about the patient may be ascertained, for example, by a nurse in the outpatient department who will not encounter the patient again and who does not necessarily know where the patient will be treated or who to pass this on to. This scenario is repeated time and again, with each successive nurse starting from scratch in the nursing process. An opportunity for avoiding this is to consider the use of notes which the patient keeps and takes from one place to another. This would seem logical in that the patient is at the centre of the process, rather than having multiple sets of notes, each at a different treatment centre. These notes need not be the full 'medical' notes, but rather a synopsis of all clinicians' input and assessment of the patient's needs, possibly with corresponding input by the patient of their understanding and thoughts about the current situation. Successive practitioners would then have an immediate synopsis of relevant information on which to base their relationship with the patient. In addition, patients would have material to refer to in order to reinforce their memory about what is happening. (Patients frequently forget information or explanations given to them for the first time and require repetition of what has been said.)

Also of great importance to patients, in terms of the continuity and significance of their care, is the multidisciplinary communication required to ensure an appropriate and smooth course of treatment and care. Nurses play a central role in advocacy and interdisciplinary communication. Understanding other professionals' priorities, treatment approaches and rationales will enable a more united and cohesive approach to patient care. Nurses receive and give essential information to or about the patient in respect of what is happening or being planned and should never underestimate the potential of their position in achieving maximum benefits for a patient.

REFERENCES

Abu-Elmagd K, Todo S, Tzakis A, Reyes J, Nour B, Furukawa H, Fung J, Demetris A, Starzl T 1994 Three years' clinical experience with intestinal transplantation. Journal of the American College of Surgeons 179(4):385–400

Bibbings J 1988 Upper gastrointestinal tract tumours. In: Tschudin V (ed.) Nursing the patient with cancer. Prentice Hall, London

Burkitt D J 1971 Epidemiology of cancer of the colon and rectum. Cancer 28:631–639

Burkitt H G, Quick C R G, Gatt D 1996 Essential surgery 2nd Edition. Churchill Livingstone, Edinburgh

Burns S J, Finlay T M D 1995 Digestive tract cancers: professional development. Nursing Times 91 (49–51) Unit 23 Parts 1–3

Chapuis P H Dixon M F Fielding L P et al 1987 Symposium of staging of colorectal cancer. International Journal of Colorectal Disease 2:123–138

Doll R, Peto R 1981 The causes of cancer. Oxford University Press, Oxford

Dukes C 1930 The spread of cancer of the rectum. British Journal of Surgery 17:643–648

Hermanek P 1989 Colorectal carcinoma: histopathological diagnosis and staging. In: Mortensen N (ed.) Colorectal cancer: Ballière's clinical gastroenterology, international practice and research. Ballière Tindall, London

Kumar V, Contran R S, Robbins S L 1992 Basic pathology, 5th edn. W B Saunders, Philadelphia

Misiewicz J J, Bartram C I, Colton P B, Mee A S, Pria A B, Thompson R P H 1988 Diseases of the colon and rectum: a guide to diagnosis. In: Gastroenterology, vol. 3. Gower Medical Publishing, London

OPCS (1992) Death statistics: series DH2, No. 19. HMSO, London

Roy C 1976 Introduction to nursing: an adaptation model. Prentice Hall, New Jersey

Souhami R, Tobias J 1995 Cancer and its management, 2nd edn. Blackwell, Oxford

Wilson J M G, Jungner G 1968 Principles and practice of screening for disease. World Health Organization, Geneva

FURTHER READING

Groenwald S L, Goodman M, Hansen Frogge M, Yarbro C H (eds) 1992 Cancer nursing: principles and practice, 2nd edn. Jones & Bartlett, Boston

Northover J, Kettner J 1992 Bowel cancer, the facts. Oxford University Press, Oxford

Sikora K, Halnan K 1990 Treatment of cancer, 2nd ed. Chapman and Hall, London

Speechley V, Rosenfield M 1996 Cancer information at your fingertips, 2nd edn. Class, London

Thomas H, Sikora K 1995 Cancer, a positive approach. Thorsons, London

USEFUL ADDRESSES

BACUP
3 Bath Place,
Rivington Street,
London,
EC2A 3JR
Freephone 0800 181199

Cancer Care Society,
21 Zetland Road,
Bristol,
BS6 7AH
0117 942 7419

Cancer Link,
17 Britannia Street,
London,
WC1X 9JN,

SCOTLAND
9 Castle Terrace,
Edinburgh,
EH1 2DP
0131 228 5557
ASIAN LANGUAGUES
(Bengali and Hindu)
0171 713 7867

Cancer Relief MacMillan Fund,
15/19 Britton Street,
London,
SW3 3TZ
0171 351 7811
*Charity funded homecare and hospital support or
financial help towards equipment for cancer patients.*

Institute for Complementary Medicine,
Register of Practitioners,
P.O. Box 194,
London,
SE16 1QZ,
0171 237 5165
*Send SAE detailing treatment area of interest
for information on reliable, relevant practitioners.*

Oesophageal Patients Association,
16 Whitfield Crescent,
Solihull,
West Midlands,
B91 3NU
0121 704 9860

Royal Marsden NHS Trust,
Haigh & Hochland Publications,
17A Ashley Road,
Cheshire,
WA15 9SP
0161 929 0190
*Patient information series booklets on
site-specific cancers.*

Palliative care

Elspeth Nesbit   Gina Copp

8

INTRODUCTION

Nursing patients in an acute care setting presents nurses with many challenges. Approximately 56% of deaths occur in acute hospitals every year (Field & James 1993). Malignant tumours of the gastrointestinal tract account for about 40,000 deaths a year in England and Wales, comprising nearly 30% of all deaths from malignant disease. Many of these patients have advanced disease at presentation (Baum et al 1993). In our experience of a busy, acute teaching hospital, patients with gastrointestinal cancers constitute one of the most common referrals for palliative care.

The stress of coping with providing care to patients with newly diagnosed and advanced malignant diseases on acute wards has been widely acknowledged (Knight & Field 1981, Field 1989, Copp & Dunn 1993). Nurses often find themselves in situations where they perceive that the skills they require in supporting patients undergoing palliative care are inadequate. For example, unlike most surgical interventions, where the likelihood of cure is the expected outcome, patients in this group will often have a limited life expectancy. Moreover, gastrointestinal diseases that bring about the need for palliative care are usually, but not exclusively, malignant. Non-malignant conditions include Crohn's disease, which can be so debilitating on some occasions as to justify referral to a palliative care support team to assist with pain and symptom management.

Although patients requiring palliative interventions present considerable challenges to all of us, the fundamental skills required to deliver such care are mostly within the scope of an experienced practitioner, provided there is an adequate support mechanism, such as the availability of a palliative care support team. Using case histories, this chapter will therefore draw on our clinical experiences to demonstrate situations in which generic and specialist nursing skills can be successfully combined to provide quality care for patients requiring palliative support for gastrointestinal conditions.

PALLIATIVE CARE AND ITS CONTRIBUTION TO GASTROINTESTINAL NURSING

The palliative care literature places particular emphasis on the importance of considering the 'whole person'. This implies the need for an integrated approach to the management of problems across a broad spectrum of treatment and care. Physical symptoms may be complex and, sometimes, intractable. Psychological and emotional difficulties can be equally challenging. The confrontation with mortality which these patients and their families face raises many questions about living as well as dying. Thus, sensitivity to the philosophical, spiritual, social and cultural dimensions of serious illness is as essential as attention to the physical manifestations. This requires a well-articulated, interdisciplinary approach, based on mutual respect amongst team members and a strong commitment to cooperation and communication. Within this model of care, the patient is encouraged to be an active participant in decision-making.

The contribution of nursing towards research in palliative care is considerable (Wilson-Barnet & Richardson 1993). Notable examples pertaining to symptom management include studies in areas such as the nature and impact of pain (Raiman 1988), mouth care (Holmes 1991, Krishnasamy 1995) and pressure area care (Walding & Andrews 1995). Insights into the specialist clinical component of the nurse's role in palliative care, particularly in relation to psychological needs, include exploratory and interpretative studies, such as those by Fleming et al (1987), Davies & O'Berle (1990) and Degner et al (1991). Copp & Dunn's (1993) study investigated the comparative frequency and complexity of symptoms across a range of acute, hospice and community settings in palliative care practice. These authors found that pain management is a key issue for nurses working in acute settings, indicating possible deficits in knowledge about pain. Both acute and community nurses identified problems associated with team relationships. Concerns relating to the shortcomings of the acute care environment, particularly to the lack of privacy for dying patients and their families, were highlighted.

These findings are of particular relevance to a focus on palliative care for people with gastrointestinal illness, where much of the care is centred on an acute ward. Here, there may be an emphasis on repeated radiological and endoscopic investigations, together with surgical intervention. The patient is often faced with a succession of hospital admissions, such as for a sequence of laser treatments for cancer of the oesophagus. A further common example is the incidence of recurrent episodes of intestinal obstruction in advancing large bowel malignancy, often precipitating the need for intermittent hospital-based care. In such circumstances, the emphasis inevitably tends to be on technical, investigative procedures, together with the ubiquitous pressures on acute beds. This creates an environment in which it is extremely difficult to provide the time, space, privacy and tranquillity conducive to comfort and the alleviation of anxiety for both patients and their families. Therefore, it is often these conditions, rather than a lack of professional nursing skills, which form barriers to good palliative care in the acute setting. Thus, skilled and experienced acute care nurses tend to compare their level of expertise unfavourably with that provided by their colleagues in specialist environments, such as a hospice.

All nurses are potentially able to give good palliative care, depending on their level of skill and experience. Palliative care is not a separate entity, but part of the continuum of generic nursing care, where episodes of acute care may be integrated within an overall framework that is essentially palliative. Alternatively, for a largely acutely managed illness, the need for specific palliative care skills for problems such as pain and symptom management or help with psychological distress may come relatively late. Much will depend on the individual patient and the particular circumstances. However, one valid generalisation is the patient's need for information regarding what help is available, both in hospital and at home. This provision requires an acknowledgement that the patient really is an individual, capable of taking charge of many aspects of decision-making. In this way, all patients are provided with equitable access to appropriate information and support, regardless of the pressurised pace of the hospital environment.

Accordingly, it should be recognised that the specialist skills of the gastroenterological nurse on the acute ward are equally important, as part of a diverse range of skills, as those of the specialist palliative care nurse and the generic community nurses in providing both comprehensive and continuous care. This combination of diverse, yet complementary knowledge and skills is crucial for the successful care of the patient and the provision of adequate support for families. The subsequent sections will focus, firstly, on some common issues relating to palliative care management of gastroenterological problems and, secondly, on the application of some of the palliative care principles in gastroenterology nursing. Case histories of practice in this field will be used to illustrate some of the common yet very challenging situations that are encountered in everyday practice.

COMMON ISSUES RELATING TO THE PALLIATIVE CARE MANAGEMENT OF GASTROENTEROLOGICAL PROBLEMS

Broadly speaking, the needs of patients requiring gastroenterology care are in the following areas:

- the management of difficult and distressing symptoms, such as pain, nausea, vomiting, nutritional difficulties, abdominal distension, constipation, respiratory problems, fatigue and insomnia
- the alleviation of psychological and emotional difficulties, such as anxiety, fear and depression.

However, these two areas should not be seen as separate entities and, indeed, there is evidence to suggest that the relief of physical symptoms can alleviate anxiety and enhance morale and, similarly, that helpful psychological intervention and social support can significantly influence physical comfort. An understanding of the complex interrelatedness of physical and psychological factors is important in the promotion of the quality of life in terminal illness.

The principal symptoms of gastrointestinal malignancy are due to obstruction of a hollow conduit, tumour bulk or blood loss. Symptoms may be acute or chronic (Baum et al 1993). Patients with gastrointestinal tumours are typically burdened with such symptoms as pain, nausea and vomiting, dysphagia, anorexia and cachexia (for review, see Doyle et al 1993). It is common to find surgical intervention forming a significant part of treatment in gastroenterological malignancy. A patient undergoing palliative surgery may, therefore, experience:

- significant debility pre-operatively through weight loss, eating difficulties, nausea and vomiting, constipation, general weakness or cachexia, anaemia and urinary problems
- prolonged recovery compared with other surgical patients through delayed wound healing or the need for nutritional support (e.g. total parenteral nutrition) and increased susceptibility to oral problems, such as candidiasis, xerostomia (dryness of the mouth), aphthous ulcers and altered taste sensation
- increased risk of wound, respiratory and urinary tract infections
- body image problems and sexual difficulties, e.g. associated with the formation of a stoma or a gastrostomy or profound weight loss
- very short-lived relief of symptoms (or less complete than was hoped for), even a short spell in hospital may be very onerous for the patient who has a limited life expectancy and longs to be at home
- an inability, due to being too ill, to participate actively in decision-making about surgical intervention.

Palliation may also involve the use of stents, as in pancreatic and oesophageal tumours, to create an artificial lumen, where there is inoperable obstruction caused by tumour resulting in, for instance, dysphagia (oesophageal cancer) or biliary obstruction (secondary to pancreatic cancer or cholangiocarcinoma). In the case of biliary obstruction, surgical bypass or non-operative stenting (percutaneous or endoscopic) of the malignant stricture provides effective palliation. Surgical bypass is usually carried out by performing either a cholecystojejunostomy or a choledochojejunostomy (Bain & Minuk 1993). These treatments may relieve symptoms for only relatively short periods. However, the attainment of such short-term gains may make an invaluable contribution to the quality of life of a patient with advanced disease.

A further procedure to be considered in gastroenterology is the formation of a venting gastrostomy or jejunostomy, described as a method of relieving nausea and vomiting for patients with inoperable intestinal obstruction as an alternative to nasogastric drainage (Baines 1993). The tube may be introduced by endoscopic means, at laparotomy or percutaneously under radiological guidance, presenting few additional problems for patients. Some patients with gastrointestinal malignancy have advanced disease at the time of diagnosis. Others return with a recurrence of tumour or metastatic disease after an interval of being well following initial surgical intervention. Commonly, intestinal obstruction, indicating a recurrence of tumour activity, is heralded by such precipitating symptoms as constipation, intractable nausea and vomiting.

The recurrence of malignancy can be very different from the time of initial diagnosis in terms of psychosocial impact (Mahon 1991). In such situations, there is a particular need for close liaison with the community team, since episodes of hospital care may alternate with periods of care at home, and a sense of continuity may help to buffer any negative consequences for the patient. Occasionally, palliative radiotherapy or chemotherapy may be combined with surgery. Treatments here are designed to minimise side-effects and disturbance to the patient's lifestyle. Kearsley (1994) describes an holistic approach in palliative chemotherapy where there is ideally a 'healing partnership' between doctor, patient and family. Nurses are well placed to develop therapeutic relationships with the patient in this kind of situation through careful assessment of needs, specifically for information, for practical help and for psychological or emotional care. Additionally, the nurse's role in establishing effective liaison within and across teams involved in the patient's care in hospital, hospice and community settings is crucial. This patient group may face a wide range of both physical and psychological difficulties during the course of an unpredictable and often profoundly debilitating illness, with episodes of home-based care alternating with those spent in hospital or in a hospice. In the following case histories, it is hoped to demonstrate and discuss some of the issues that may arise within a collaborative palliative care approach.

Managing difficult symptoms in advanced illness (refer to Case history 8.1)

The management of symptoms requires a logical and thorough approach with attention directed towards teasing out individual problems which, in turn, are seen as interlinking parts of a whole picture, which is the unique experience of the patient. Patients with gastrointestinal cancers frequently achieve a remission period following initial treatment in which life returns to 'normal'. A recurrence may therefore represent a profound psychosocial threat (Mahon 1991). Mahon draws attention to a lack of research into how patients cope with recurrence and suggests that an understanding of the patient's previous experience of illness, treatment and contact with the health care system is important in planning nursing intervention, to help patients and their families with the new crisis which recurrence brings.

The recurrence of illness in gastrointestinal malignancy may be associated with the gradual or more sudden onset of such symptoms as pain, nausea, vomiting, dehydration, anorexia, constipation and intestinal obstruction. The medical management of these symptoms may involve surgical or pharmacological intervention. Typical features of this kind of situation are the patient's extreme debility as a result of symptoms and/or surgery, and a strong wish to return home. For Anne, fighting the illness and pursuing all treatment options was almost instinctive. So, too, was her determination to return home as soon as possible to be in her own home with her family.

Intestinal obstruction is caused by an occlusion to the lumen or a lack of

---

Case history 8.1

Anne underwent a series of surgical bypass procedures to control an incurable primary bowel tumour. Her symptoms included pain, nausea and vomiting. These symptoms had been well-controlled at home for a time. Discussion of the likely future course of her disease had not been encouraged by Anne or her family at her first meeting with the team. Throughout her illness, her main source of strength was the indefatigable support of her family and her strong religious faith.

It was difficult to know whether her determination to fight her disease was prompted by a sense of commitment to her family, for whom she appeared to have a special role as the 'fulcrum' of all their lives, religious conviction that this was the 'right thing to do', or simply a strong instinct to continue to fight passionately for life. It may simply have been a combination of all three.

On a subsequent admission to hospital, her symptoms were abdominal pain, nausea and vomiting, dehydration, constipation and considerable distress. Her acute symptoms were brought under control over the next 24 h by increasing her opioid analgesia, adjusting her anti-emetic therapy and instituting intravenous fluids, since she was unable to tolerate oral fluids. Her anxiety appeared to diminish, partly in response to the pharmacological intervention and partly because, as she said, she felt 'safe' in hospital.

This feeling of security may have been helped by the fact that she had returned to a familiar ward, where she felt at ease with, and trusted, the staff and where she knew her family could visit at any time. They needed to be with Anne as much as she welcomed their presence. It was as if some intangible web of support remained intact while they maintained this vigil, with a mutual exchange of strength and love. In fact, it was sometimes difficult to ensure that Anne had sufficient rest and sleep.

Subsequently, Anne opted to undergo a further palliative bypass procedure to relieve the recurrent bowel obstruction. She was already very weak and the limited prospects of success had been discussed carefully with her and with her family. Surgery was successful and Anne made a good recovery and returned home, where she continued to be with her family, while she slowly deteriorated over the succeeding weeks.

---

normal propulsion which prevents or delays intestinal contents from passing along the gastrointestinal tract. The incidence of bowel obstruction is a common event in patients with abdominal or pelvic cancers, with a prevalence of between 4.4 and 24% in people with colorectal cancer (Ripamonti 1994). Intestinal obstruction may present acutely with the sudden onset of colicky, abdominal pain, vomiting and constipation, or may follow a more gradual, insidious pattern. The level of obstruction will also determine the presence of particular clinical features:

• *Distension* is the most early constant and continuing sign of obstruction and is associated particularly with large bowel lesions (Twycross & Lack 1986)

• *Vomiting* is more prominent in obstructions of the stomach, duodenum and jejunum and tends to be a less frequent or later development in large bowel obstruction (Baines et al 1985, Twycross & Lack 1986, Ripamonti 1994).

• *Pain* may be present due to abdominal distension, tumour mass, hepatomegaly or abdominal colic in small and large bowel obstruction (Ripamonti 1994). Symptoms may gradually worsen, but may be intermittent or spontaneously resolve, even without treatment (Baines 1993).

Pain

A commitment to effective pain management is a central tenet of palliative care. Pain is a complex phenomenon. Its presence provides no concrete evidence for the observer. A haemorrhage, a bout of vomiting, a fit or lapse into unconsciousness all indicate that something serious is happening. When someone experiences pain, helpful intervention will depend as much upon listening to and believing the information provided by the sufferer as upon the therapist's knowledge of analgesia. Pain may herald an undiagnosed event or be the consequence of it. The perception of pain by the person experiencing it will also be influenced by such factors as fear, apprehension, anxiety, depression, environmental circumstances, cultural conditioning and previous painful experiences.

Copp & Dunn's (1993) study of nurses' perceptions of frequent and difficult problems in hospital, hospice and community settings indicated that pain was one of the two most frequently encountered problems, and the most difficult in the acute setting. Paice et al (1991) found that pain management was inadequate in the postoperative period in a study of 34 patients on a surgical oncology ward. The authors concluded that deficiencies in assessment and documentation of individual patients' pain was a problem, despite the availability of appropriate analgesia. The patient in pain on the acute ward needs to feel sure that his or her story will be listened to and acted upon promptly. Some key factors are:

• The circumstances precipitating admission to hospital may be crucial indicators of the nature and significance of the pain, e.g.:

— has the same kind of pain been experienced before?
— how long had the pain been present prior to admission?
— what other symptoms have accompanied the pain?
— is the pain continuous or intermittent?
— are one or more pains present?
— precise nature and location of the pain – what is the pain like?
— has anything helped the pain?
— has anything made it worse?
— are there any specific concerns regarding the implications of the pain?

• The management of pain depends on thorough and determined assessment. This involves knowledge, competence and confidence in the use of appropriate pharmacology, including:

— an understanding of the principles determining the use of both non-opioid and opioid analgesia and the titration of analgesic medication in relation to the individual patient's experience of pain

— knowledge of the side-effects of opioid analgesia, i.e. nausea and vomiting and constipation, so that appropriate prophylactic anti-emetics and laxatives can be prescribed
— an understanding of non-pharmacological interventions which may be helpful alongside analgesia, e.g. special beds, heat pads, cold packs, massage, relaxation exercises, listening and counselling skills
— effective interdisciplinary communication and cooperation, ensuring effective use of specialist expertise
— regular review of pain relief once intervention has been decided upon.

The need for an adjustment of the dose of analgesia should be anticipated in the light of factors such as the origin and nature of the pain, the stage of the disease process and any concurrent treatment.

The use of a pain tool may be helpful, such as a visual analogue scale, a verbal rating scale or a pain chart, e.g. the McGill Pain Questionnaire (Melzack & Wall 1983) or The London Hospital Pain Observation Chart (Raiman 1988).

Pain cannot simply be attributed to the amount of tissue damage that is evident. This principle will apply in any situation. In palliative care situations, the patient may associate the onset of pain with advancing illness and, in the case of malignant disease, pain is often experienced by the patient as a reminder of mortality.

In the acute setting of a specialist gastroenterology ward, the patient undergoing surgery for an intestinal obstruction may not be facing a technically difficult procedure, but is confronted with the inevitability of progressive disease and, perhaps, the possibility of a disfiguring procedure (e.g. if a stoma is likely to be necessary). This may create new concerns about the implications for important personal relationships, further curtailment of independence and, thus, an overall threat to quality of life. Such a patient is also likely to be constantly reminded of the rapid recovery of fellow patients, perhaps undergoing surgery for non-malignant conditions.

It is therefore essential that nursing care for such patients includes pain assessment on admission/pre-operatively and postoperatively. The pre-operative level of analgesia will have to be reviewed in the light of surgical intervention, but residual cancer pain may continue to be a factor in the need for postoperative analgesia. If a thorough assessment of pain is made prior to surgical intervention, good pain relief postoperatively will be facilitated. Clear and careful communication between nursing and medical colleagues, including the anaesthetic team, is essential.

Following surgery and discharge home, Anne needed subcutaneous morphine for abdominal pain and an anti-emetic acting directly on the vomiting centre (cyclizine) to control nausea, via a portable syringe driver. She was readmitted to the ward when her symptoms worsened and hyoscine butyl-bromide was added to her infusion to combat the onset of colicky pain which often accompanies bowel obstruction. With this drug combination and the support of her GP, district nurse and community Macmillan nurse, Anne was able to spend the final few weeks of her life at home, much weaker, but with her symptoms controlled.

The use of portable syringe drivers in palliative care

A portable syringe driver can be used to deliver drugs over a 24-h period subcutaneously, when the oral route is compromised. Indications for considering this approach include:

- difficulty in swallowing
- intractable nausea or vomiting
- intestinal obstruction (where absorption will be unreliable and vomiting may be a concurrent problem)
- weakness or diminished level of consciousness making administration of oral medication impracticable.

Drugs which may be administered subcutaneously in this way include opioid analgesics (morphine or diamorphine), certain anti-emetics, antispasmodics (hyoscine butylbromide for colicky pain) and sedatives (for instance, midazolam). Careful conversion of opioids from an oral to parenteral dose must be ensured (Twycross 1995), and provision must also be made for giving an appropriate 'breakthrough' dose if required (this can also be given subcutaneously; it can be helpful to consider an additional subcutaneous 'butterfly' line for the purpose).

Advantages of using subcutaneous infusions

- Removes need for painful, intramuscular injections
- Small and portable and therefore acceptable to ambulant patients
- Small volume of fluid administered – usually no more than 10–20 ml over 24 h
- The patient can be cared for at home with a similar pump.

Psychological care for a profoundly weak patient (refer to Case history 8.1)

Weakness is commonly one of the most pervasive and indefinable symptoms of a serious illness. Moreover, it may be viewed as either a symptom or as a natural consequence of advancing illness. It is hard for a weak and debilitated person to discuss the possibility or the proximity of dying, but it may be a crucial factor in either mitigating or compounding the patient's experience of suffering. To avoid recognising the need to discuss this and facilitating the opportunity to do so can only deepen the distress for the patient who wishes to discuss these issues. Equally, it is not appropriate to make an assumption that every patient will find this therapeutic. The expression of a preference may depend on an individual's coping mechanism, so that avoidance or denial may be an instrumental part in that person's capacity to manage what is happening. For some, it may simply be a matter of conserving precious energy. De Montigny (1993) noted that:

> the priority for terminal patients is the preservation of their remaining supply of physical energy for the simple act of survival; they do not want to waste it on the exploration of their emotional world.

This kind of situation requires us to be able to make some kind of judgement based on an accurate understanding of the patient's needs and wishes. We need to be able to assess the psychological as well as the physical status of the patient and to recognise these factors as interdependent. Thus, psychological care should be a component of the nursing care plan for any patient, so that such care can be planned to anticipate potential needs and problems, rather that being a reactive intervention (Nichols 1993). Eliciting the most helpful strategy in a scenario such as that described in Anne's case can be particularly exacting, because it involves close monitoring of both the patient's capacity and their desire to explain and explore feelings and worries, as Montigny (1993) suggests. In palliative care, such a situation may change from day to day and therefore will require regular assessment and review.

However, the underlying principles apply to any nursing situation where an assessment has to be made about a patient's capacity at specific times during illness to engage in an exploration of anxieties or concerns about the future. All nurses will have acquired some skill in assessing and interpreting the links between the physical and psychological symptoms experienced by the individual patient. A specialist nursing knowledge of gastroenterology will therefore represent an essential contribution to palliative as well as acute nursing care.

Promoting autonomy and control (refer to Case history 8.2)

The nurse's role in supporting the patient's desire for the preservation of

---

Case history 8.2

Molly was readmitted to hospital a few months following surgical resection of a cancer of the colon. The symptoms of nausea, abdominal pain and constipation had returned. Further surgery proved impossible, and chemotherapy was discussed with her as a palliative attempt to improve symptoms and prognosis.

Her symptoms had improved with analgesic, anti-emetic and laxative medication and, although she felt weak and could eat very little, she had resolved to cope by adopting a defiant approach to her illness, taking a positive view of treatment, and by making all the arrangements for her own funeral. She was determined that her relationships with family and friends should be unclouded by reticence, embarrassment and fear, and she clearly recognised that she would have to take the lead in this respect.

Molly's expressed need was for information across a range of subjects. What might happen to her body as she became more ill? How could she conserve energy to cope with the chemotherapy and, at the same time, support her family? There were also a number of very practical concerns, such as obtaining a wheelchair, as walking was becoming more and more difficult. All this was communicated with great clarity; her emotion was not hidden, but she wanted to gather her resources, like armour for battle, and not be engulfed in an 'empathic blanket'.

independence through the crisis of illness is crucial. When a full recovery is expected, this process can be expected to take the form of a linear progression and therefore be reasonably straightforward. However, when illness results in some permanent alteration in health or an impairment of independence, the concept of recovery will be more ambivalent and complex, with an emphasis on rehabilitation, adjustment and coping.

Case history 8.2 illustrates how people who are ill can, nonetheless, be strongly motivated to retain control of their lives. It is important that we understand this as a right, not a privilege. Compliance with treatment or care should not render the individual a hostage to the therapeutic team as well as to the illness. The question of the nature of the nurse's role in promoting autonomy was highlighted by the recurrence of this theme during this episode of care. It seemed that Molly's needs were twofold:

• Firstly, she had a need for specific, accurate information. This would enable her to plan for the future, albeit a very limited future. She knew very well that her own professional skills were those of a problem-solver, which she felt she could use to help her, provided that she had clear information and that other people were open and honest with her.

• The second priority seemed to be to convey an assurance that she would be treated as an autonomous, unique individual; an affirmation that serious and debilitating illness would not result in patronising or prescriptive attitudes.

The social support literature provides us with some clear guidelines in the area of information-giving. For instance, Dunkel-Schetter's (1984) research indicates the importance of providing the right amount of information to the patient and that it should come from an expert. Dunkel-Schetter et al (1987) evolved a three-category classification of social support: emotional support, informational support and instrumental assistance to assess the needs of the individual patient in this respect.

In Molly's case, the need for information was crucial, as she herself emphasised. There was also a limited need for instrumental assistance, for example, about how to acquire equipment such as a wheelchair. The need for emotional support was more difficult to assess, especially since the team's contact with Molly was over a period of 3 days only, but it was clear she looked to her family for this, and from us sought only a professional acknowledgement of her feelings and the weight of what she was experiencing. Assessment, planning and evaluation are as important in giving psychological care as they are in giving physical care (Nichols 1993).

During conversations with members of the team, Molly generally took the lead in directing the content, the pace and the duration of each interaction. Although she was in fact already very ill, she had firm ideas about what she needed to accomplish. She may have sensed that her illness might overtake her before these goals were attained, but she indicated that her need to concentrate on living was of fundamental importance to her. Individual patients react differently in these circumstances. A decision to defy an overwhelming illness may be mistaken for denial of its seriousness. It should be recognised that goals and hopes exist on a sliding scale. Denial of an ominous symptom or loss of strength often suggests a protective coping mechanism, rather than a real lack of insight. The nurse's ability to understand and work with the subtlety and complexity of a changing and unpredictable situation may help both the patient and family members to adjust to a progressive and often frightening process as the patient becomes weaker and more dependent.

Discharge planning (refer to Case history 8.2)

Here the roles of the primary nurse, who has overall responsibility for planning the patient's nursing care, and the specialist palliative care nurse can be seen as distinct yet complementary. The patient's stay in an acute hospital is relatively short and focused principally on resolving or alleviating the physical manifestations of illness. The recognition of additional needs, in particular in relation to planning continuity of care when the patient goes home, is an important part of the primary nurse's role. Key channels of communication are those between the primary or team nurse and the community nurse. Patients with gastrointestinal conditions frequently need follow-up assessment and care for surgical, or sometimes fungating, wounds, assistance with stoma management, dietary advice and, in addition, help with emotional adjustment to an advancing illness.

The role of the specialist palliative care nurse in discharge planning may include discussion with the patient regarding referral to a specialist community service, such as a Macmillan team or the possible implications of further treatment. Families who are about to take on the care of a seriously ill patient at home sometimes have recollections of, or fears about, traumatic circumstances surrounding the dying process, and it may help them to explore these and seek reassurance regarding particular concerns. In Molly's case, the important questions about continuing care related to the possible side-effects of impending chemotherapy and her wish to establish early contact with the hospice. In response to the latter, an informal visit to the hospice was arranged as part of the immediate follow-up care upon discharge home.

Working with different levels of awareness (refer to Case history 8.3)

Glaser & Strauss (1965) identified four awareness contexts in reflecting the degree to which patients with terminal illness were aware of this reality. According to this framework, the first level or 'closed awareness context' is one in which the patient is deprived of any explicit confirmation of his or her condition. In a 'suspicion awareness context', the patient guesses the prognosis, but is not directly informed, and is thus tacitly denied the opportunity to discuss fears and worries openly. In a situation of 'mutual pretence', there is a reciprocal pretence that the patient is not going to die, although patient and staff all know otherwise. The open acknowledgement of imminent death occurs only when the context is one of 'open awareness'. The issue of awareness is a complex one, particularly in the setting of the acute surgical ward (Knight & Field 1981). For example, a poor prognosis or outcome following surgery may have to be withheld for several days until the patient is well

---

Case history 8.3

Jim had cancer of the colon and there had been hope of surgery to remove a single liver metastasis. A laparotomy revealed that the liver involvement was widespread and therefore inoperable. These findings were explained to Jim and his wife and palliative chemotherapy was considered.

Referral to the palliative care support team was felt by Jim to be premature, but his wife welcomed the opportunity to discuss and plan future care and support. Jim's wife knew him to be reserved and independent – aware of the implications of unsuccessful surgery, but unwilling to allow anyone to make an issue of this. However, she knew that they would both need help to manage later on and recognised that they had different coping styles.

On the day of discharge home, Jim expressed his reservation about offers of help at that time but, in fact, he indicated a clear understanding of what lay ahead and discussed many issues, ranging from practical concerns to anxieties about anticipated symptoms and concerns for his family and future lifestyle. His priority at that time was not to abdicate his sense of responsibility towards his family.

---

enough to receive bad news. This has implications for what news any relatives may be given in the intervening time. A difficulty here can arise if relatives wish to continue to 'protect' the patient from reality beyond the initial recovery period.

In Jim's case there was complete understanding of the implications of failed surgery, but he chose not to explore this in detail with the palliative care support team. However, he was able to talk about his situation more easily with the nurses who were involved in his daily care. This may have been because their expertise involved monitoring closely his recovery from surgery alongside an assessment of his psychological care needs. The palliative care support team may have represented a future Jim was not yet ready to consider. Jim's wife expressed her understanding of this and, whilst seeking support for herself, she respected Jim's wish not to explore his feelings at the time. Thus, this scenario demonstrates that patients may choose with whom they talk and the extent of the disclosure. Clearly, it is crucial to be aware of and to respect the patient's choice and to understand that the patient's decision may change at a future time.

A significant number of patients undergo gastrointestinal surgery with a reasonable hope of a curative procedure, while the surgical options in reality turn out to be a palliative bypass procedure or simply an 'open and close' procedure. This scenario is tough for everyone involved. A good recovery from the operation itself can seem like a parody of the surgical experience of the other patients with acute conditions, who can expect a swift and full recovery. In such difficult circumstances, the manner of imparting information and the preparation for giving the patient bad and upsetting news are critically important. The nursing skills needed in such situations are essentially good communication skills which should be part of any qualified nurse's repertoire. This was clearly applicable in Jim's case. However, research has shown that poor communication with patients may persist even after specialist education (Wilkinson 1991), and that such communication problems have negative implications for the support of both relatives and staff. Faulkner (1992) identifies some barriers to effective assessment in the nurse–patient interaction as 'closed' and 'leading' questions, 'making assumptions', 'distancing' and the fear of unleashing strong emotions. She suggests that problem identification through careful assessment will help towards setting goals which are relevant and achievable for the individual patient.

Supporting the family (refer to Case history 8.3)

In Jim's case, it became clear very early on, at the first meeting with him and his wife together, that he did not, at that point, wish to talk about his illness or the future. He wanted to concentrate on getting stronger after an operation which had not brought the hoped-for outcome; he needed time to gather his thoughts and his strength. This would be helped by nursing directed positively at physical recovery, relief of pain and the promotion of comfort. Jim's wife, however, was already thinking about what lay ahead and she needed to lay some foundation plans for that time.

These differing needs were discussed at length with Jim's primary nurse and other members of the nursing and medical teams and a shared care plan evolved. The primary nurse and her colleagues continued to assume full responsibility for Jim's nursing care; the role of the specialist nurse here was more peripheral – the discussion of pain and symptoms, keeping up to date with postoperative progress and how Jim was feeling. The specialist nursing contribution was perhaps, in the first place, the recognition and affirmation of the differing needs of two partners, who, despite their closeness, were coping at a differing pace with what was happening at a critical moment in Jim's illness. The team continued to see Jim's wife almost daily throughout this period of about a week. Her understanding of the discrepancy in their apparent levels of awareness was very clearly articulated. She knew that, at that moment, Jim needed to be optimistic, yet understood him well enough to perceive his underlying comprehension of his real prognosis.

Hydration and feeding in palliative care (refer to Case history 8.4)

At the same time as sustaining hope for Ian, it was also important to pay similar attention to his physical care. This had involved parenteral feeding following his surgery. The closeness to surgical intervention of other palliative treatments highlights the paradoxical nature of giving palliative care in the acute setting. The team's experience suggests that, increasingly, decisions about commencing or continuing hydration and feeding are profoundly difficult to make. Copp & Dunn (1993) found that concerns about patient nutrition (alongside pain) were the most frequently occurring problems experienced across the hospice, hospital and community settings sampled in their survey.

Ian appeared emaciated and weak and was described as cachectic. 'Cancer

---

Case history 8.4

Ian had undergone palliative bypass surgery to relieve an obstruction by cancer at the head of the pancreas. He was extremely weak and cachectic; parenteral feeding had been commenced to alleviate this. It now seemed unlikely that the outcome of surgery would be a successful restoration of oral hydration and nutrition.

Ian had hoped to join his family on a holiday – which he knew would be his last. When this began to seem impossible, he restructured this hope around a plan to leave the hospital and be at home with his family, who lived some distance away. He knew that he was dying and seemed not to resent that this death would be premature (he was in his 40s) – only desiring that it should not be in hospital, an institution where he felt trapped.

A plan was evolved with Ian to arrange his transfer to a hospice close to his family's home. His capacity to participate in this was limited and unpredictable. His awareness of his predicament was, nonetheless, quite clear, although he alluded to it only indirectly.

On one occasion, the poignancy of this awareness was communicated without words. The patient in the next bed was recovering from surgery. The evidence for this was obvious – the lively exchanges with a succession of visitors and enjoyment of the cricket match on the television. Ian was barely conscious. He listened to the conversations around him and smiled. His eyes closed and he drifted off to sleep again. After this, his eyes barely opened again. Over the next 24 h he became weaker and the plans never came to fruition. This situation remains a powerful one, for it demonstrated that while Ian appeared to be accepting his dying 'peacefully', he seemed at the same time aware of the irony of the contrast between his imminent death and the normal recovery of his fellow patients.

---

cachexia syndrome' is an ill-defined phenomenon. It is a term used to describe weight loss, muscle wasting and anorexia. It is likely that such weight loss results from an alteration in food metabolism caused by tumour necrosis factor (cachexin) produced by the tumour. Reduced desire and capacity to eat are normal consequences in advanced disease (Boyd & Beeken 1994). These authors also point out that the nutritional intake of patients receiving tube feeds, such as through gastrostomy or jejunostomy tubes, is no longer controlled by a physiological or psychological drive to eat. It is therefore important that the patient's wishes with regard to nutritional support are respected. In some cases, it may be difficult for family members to come to terms with the cessation or reduction of nutritional support, since feeding has strong cultural connections with the expression of nurturing and caring. This may be expressed in the home setting where families often persevere to tempt or persuade a reluctant patient to eat. Of course, these problems are not confined to patients with primary gastrointestinal malignant disease, since gastrointestinal symptoms are prevalent in all far-advanced cancers (Dunlop 1989, Copp & Dunn 1993).

Ian was fed via a central line and this continued until the day before he died. Fortunately, in this case, the issue of hydration and nutrition was not an area of contention for him or the team caring for him on the ward. However, the issue of hydration in advanced illness can be controversial and problematic. There is a growing body of literature debating the benefits and burdens of continued hydration in advanced disease. Sutcliffe & Holmes (1994) have provided a useful review of the literature and advocate wider discussion of an issue which is crucial to patient comfort and quality of life in palliative care. A particular consequence of dehydration is dry mouth (Twycross & Lichter 1993, Sutcliffe & Holmes 1994).

Mouth care

Mouth care is an area where nursing has a significant role to play, particularly in oral assessment. In advanced disease, the most common problems are a coated mouth and tongue, a dry mouth (leading to a very distressing perception of thirst), altered taste, pain and infection (Krishnasamy 1995). The literature suggests that the frequency of mouth care is more important than the cleansing agents used. There is only anecdotal evidence for the efficacy of many agents commonly used in mouth care, and some can cause pain and alter the alkaline pH of saliva. A small, soft toothbrush may be best for plaque removal from teeth, while foam sticks are a more gentle treatment if the mouth is painful or likely to bleed. Krishnasamy (1995) suggested dilute hydrogen peroxide (a solution of 15 ml to 200 ml of water for badly coated mouths and tongues), but warns that this solution should be mixed just before use and should not be continued once the condition begins to improve as new tissue may be damaged. Candidiasis and bacterial infections should be promptly identified and treated. Additionally, an imaginative approach to diet and the inclusion of plain or flavoured ice cubes, varied fluids, crushed fruit and saliva substitutes may also be helpful.

The meaning of hope in palliative care (refer to Case history 8.4)

The concept of hope within palliative care is paradoxical and challenging. For example, as in Ian's case, it may be difficult to comprehend the resilience and fortitude expressed in an individual's ability to sustain hope in the face of limited life-expectancy and the physical or emotional pain that accompanies this prospect. The evidence of hope in such circumstances may therefore be ascribed to 'denial' or to an extreme form of spiritual resilience. Weisman (1979) equated 'hoping' with 'coping', i.e. a character trait, rather than a strategy. Herth (1990) found that hope was present in terminally ill people, despite their physical limitations or nearness to death, based on aspects of 'being' rather than rational expectations. This, too, suggests that part of the crisis of mortality involves a spiritual dimension that we should be aware of and respond to, even if it is an intensely personal and potentially incommunicable experience.

Herth's research suggests that the presence of a caring relationship is of critical importance in sustaining hope. Hockley (1993) also defines hope as transcending expectation and suggests that nurses can play a role in contributing to either hope or hopelessness in patients. Consequently, it appears that hope can be experienced independently of hope for recovery or cure. 'Finding meaning' may be one example of this, since it appears that suffering does not necessarily extinguish hope. The phenomenon of 'hope' in this context is a clear reminder of the complex interrelatedness of physical and psychological factors in palliative care, and represents a considerable challenge to any member of the therapeutic team. Accordingly, the capacity of the individual to make sense of, or gain some mastery of, this most demanding and daunting human experience should never be underestimated.

Caring for Ian was thus challenging in a number of ways in relation to giving hope. He was a young person who still hoped to regain some independence. Throughout the few days of the final stage of his illness, his hope to be independent of an institutional setting was adjusted to hoping to be cared for by his family or in a hospice, then, finally, to a realisation that he would probably die in hospital. This kind of situation typifies an area of nursing care that requires both honesty and sensitive listening skills, avoiding the temptation to give false hope and yet not taking away what might be possible. Often this involves the nurse in using professional knowledge which will permit an element of risk-taking, negotiating the patient's potential, personal goals and aspirations and providing sustained support if the situation changes.

CONCLUSION

This chapter has highlighted the specialist and generic skills that are crucial to the successful support of patients requiring palliative care in gastroenterological settings. The case histories have shown the common, yet very challenging, situations that are encountered in everyday nursing practice. Clearly, each situation is unique to the individuals concerned and is seldom clear-cut. Increasingly, medical and surgical innovations have extended treatment possibilities for patients in the advanced stages of both malignant and nonmalignant illnesses. Nursing has a significant contribution to make in recognising the challenge and complexity of the needs of such patients and their carers, and in contributing imaginatively and sensitively to a plan of care which can make a positive difference within the limitations of advanced illness.

REFERENCES

Bain V G, Minuk G Y 1993 Jaundice, ascites and hepatic encephalopathy. In: Doyle D, Hanks G W C, MacDonald N (eds) Oxford textbook of palliative medicine. Oxford University Press, Oxford, p 337–348
Baines M 1993 The pathophysiology and management of malignant intestinal obstruction. In: Doyle D, Hanks G W C, MacDonald N (eds) Oxford textbook of palliative medicine. Oxford University Press, Oxford, p 311–316
Baines M, Oliver D J, Carter R L 1985 Medical management of intestinal obstruction in patients with advanced malignant disease. Lancet, November 3: Vol 2:991–993
Baum M, Breach N M, Shepherd J H, Shearer R J, Meirion Thomas J, Ball A 1993 Surgical palliation. In: Doyle D, Hanks G W C, MacDonald N (eds) Oxford textbook of palliative medicine. Oxford University Press, Oxford, p 129–140

Boyd K J, Beeken L 1994 Tube feeding in palliative care. Palliative Medicine 8:156–158

Copp G, Dunn G 1993 Frequent and difficult problems perceived by nurses caring for the dying in community, hospice and acute care settings. Palliative Medicine 7:19–25

Davies B, O'Berle K 1990 Dimensions of the supportive role of the nurse in palliative care. Oncology Nursing Forum 17 (1):87–94

Degner L F, Gow C M, Thompson L A 1991 Critical nursing behaviours in care for the dying. Cancer Nursing 14(5):246–253

De Montigny J 1993 Distress, stress and solidarity in palliative care. Omega 27(1):5–15

Doyle D, Hanks G W C, MacDonald N (eds) 1993 Gastrointestinal Symptoms. Oxford textbook of palliative medicine. Oxford University Press, Oxford, p 282–348

Dunkel-Schetter C 1984 Social support and cancer: findings based on patient interviews and their implications. Journal of Social Issues 40 (4):77–98

Dunkel-Schetter C, Folkman S, Lazarus R S 1987 Correlates of social support. Journal of Personality and Social Psychology 53(1):71–80

Dunlop G M 1989 A study of the relative frequency and importance of gastrointestinal symptoms, and weakness in patients with far advanced cancer: student paper. Palliative Medicine 4:37–43

Faulkner A 1992 Effective interaction with patients. Churchill Livingstone, Edinburgh

Field D 1989 Nursing the dying. Tavistock Routledge, London

Field D, James N 1993 Where and how people die. In: Clark D (ed) The future for palliative care. Open University Press, Buckingham, p 6–29

Fleming C, Scanlon C, D'Agostino N S 1987 A study of the comfort needs of patients with advanced cancer. Cancer Nursing 10(5):237–243

Glaser B, Strauss A 1965 Awareness of dying. Aldine, Chicago

Herth K 1990 Fostering hope in the terminally ill. Journal of Advanced Nursing 15:1250–1259

Hockley J 1993 The concept of hope and the will to live. Palliative Medicine 7:181–186

Holmes S 1991 The oral complications of specific anticancer therapy. International Journal of Nursing Studies 28(4):343–360

Kearsley J H 1994 Some basic guidelines in the use of chemotherapy for patients with incurable malignancy. Palliative Medicine 8:11–17

Knight M, Field D 1981 A silent conspiracy: coping with dying cancer patients on an acute surgical ward. Journal of Advanced Nursing 6:221–229

Krishnasamy M 1995 The nurse's role in oral care. European Journal of Palliative Care 2(2):8–9

Mahon S 1991 Managing the psychosocial consequences of cancer recurrence: implications for nurses. Oncology Nursing Forum 18(3):577–583

Melzack R, Wall P 1988 The challenge of pain. Penguin, Middlesex

Nichols K 1993 Psychological care in physical illness. Chapman and Hall, London

Paice J M, Mahon S, Faut-Callahan M 1991 Factors associated with adequate pain control in hospitalized postsurgical patients diagnosed with cancer. Cancer Nursing 14(6):298–305

Raiman J 1988 Pain and its management. In: Wilson-Barnett J, Raiman J (eds) Nursing issues in research and terminal care. Basil Wiley and Sons, Chichester

Ripamonti C 1994 Management of bowel obstruction in advanced cancer. Current Opinion in Oncology 6(4):351–357

Sutcliffe J, Holmes S 1994 Dehydration: burden or benefit to the patient? Journal of Advanced Nursing 19:71–76

Twycross R G 1995 Introducing palliative care. Radcliffe Medical Press, Abingdon

Twycross R G, Lack S A 1986 Control of alimentary symptoms in far advanced cancer. Churchill Livingstone, Edinburgh

Twycross R G, Lichter I 1993 The terminal phase. In: Doyle D, Hanks G W C, MacDonald N (eds) Oxford textbook of palliative medicine. Oxford University Press, Oxford

Walding M, Andrews C 1995 Managing pressure sores in palliative care. Professional Nurse 11(1):33–38

Weisman D 1979 Coping with cancer. McGraw Hill, USA

Wilkinson S 1991 Factors which influence how nurses communicate with cancer patients. Journal of Advanced Nursing 16:677–688

Wilson-Barnett J, Richardson A 1993 Nursing research and palliative care. In: Doyle D, Hanks G W C, MacDonald N (eds) Oxford textbook of palliative medicine. Oxford University Press, Oxford, p 97–102

FURTHER READING

Barraclough J 1994 Cancer and emotion; a practical guide to psycho-oncology. John Wiley and Sons, Chichester

Buckman R 1992 How to break bad news. Papermac, London

Carroll D, Bowsher D 1993 Pain management and nursing care. Butterworth-Heinemann, Oxford

Maguire P 1985 Barriers to psychological care of the dying. British Medical Journal 291:1711–1713

Oliver D J 1988 Syringe drivers in palliative care: a review. Palliative Medicine 2:21–26

Nutrition

Helen Hamilton   Jacqueline Boorman

NUTRITIONAL SUPPORT

Malnutrition occurs when a patient is unable, or unwilling, to meet their metabolic requirements for one or more nutrients. Patients with gastrointestinal disease are a particularly vulnerable patient group, as dietary inadequacy, reduced appetites and nutrient malabsorption can all contribute to malnutrition. Neglecting the importance of nutrition could mean a delay in the patient's recovery or, worse still, it could result in a life-threatening situation.

How do people become malnourished in hospital?

Dietary inadequacy, reduced appetites and nutrient malabsorption have already been cited as reasons why the patient with a gastrointestinal disease could become malnourished, but other reasons do exist (Fig. 9.1).

Nutritional assessment

Failing to identify patients who are at risk of malnutrition is a common problem in hospitals. One of the major recommendations of the report *A positive approach to nutrition as treatment* (Kings Fund Centre 1992) was that early identification should go some way to keeping the risk of complications to a minimum. It was suggested that information about each patient's nutritional status should be mandatory in medical and nursing admission records, and that nutritional status should be regularly reviewed throughout a patient's stay in hospital. A gastroenterology nurse's role in the identification of patients at risk of malnutrition is therefore a crucial part of the nutritional assessment for the following reasons:

- nurses see patients every day
- they are available at mealtimes and are therefore able to monitor intake
- they are physically able to ensure delivery of supplements, meals, snacks, tube feeds to the patient
- they are able to encourage and support patients and their relatives

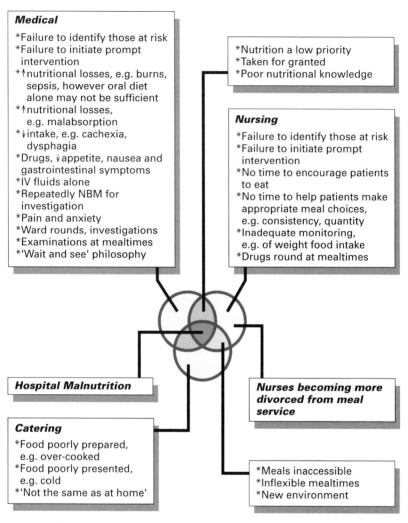

Medical
*Failure to identify those at risk
*Failure to initiate prompt
 intervention
*↑nutritional losses, e.g. burns,
 sepsis, however oral diet
 alone may not be sufficient
*↑nutritional losses,
 e.g. malabsorption
*↓intake, e.g. cachexia,
 dysphagia
*Drugs, ↓appetite, nausea and
 gastrointestinal symptoms
*IV fluids alone
*Repeatedly NBM for
 investigation
*Pain and anxiety
*Ward rounds, investigations
*Examinations at mealtimes
*'Wait and see' philosophy

*Nutrition a low priority
*Taken for granted
*Poor nutritional knowledge

Nursing
*Failure to identify those at risk
*Failure to initiate prompt
 intervention
*No time to encourage patients
 to eat
*No time to help patients make
 appropriate meal choices,
 e.g. consistency, quantity
*Inadequate monitoring,
 e.g. of weight food intake
*Drugs round at mealtimes

Hospital Malnutrition

**Nurses becoming more
divorced from meal
service**

Catering
*Food poorly prepared,
 e.g. over-cooked
*Food poorly presented,
 e.g. cold
*'Not the same as at home'

*Meals inaccessible
*Inflexible mealtimes
*New environment

Fig 9.1 Why do people become malnourished in hospital?

- they are able to refer patients to a dietitian when necessary
- they can alert doctors to the patient's nutritional status on ward rounds
  and ensure that it is not overlooked.

How do you assess?

It is important to realise that no single test used in isolation is able to identify
a malnourished patient. A number of hospitals have developed nutrition
checklists designed to help nurses identify at-risk patients, therefore preventing malnutrition. A checklist will also prompt quick initiation of nutritional

Table 9.1 Sample nutrition checklist to assess nutritional status (to be assessed on a weekly basis) (based on a checklist from the Department of Nutrition and Dietetics, Oxford Radcliffe Hospital, unpublished)

Area	Score
Appearance	
Pressure sore(s) or Waterlow score > 10	3
Obvious weight loss/cachexia	1
Muscle wasting	1
Sore mouth/tongue, affecting oral intake	1
Oedema (peripheral)	1
General neglected or unkempt appearance	1
Clinical condition	
Decreased level of consciousness	3
7 days pre- or postoperatively*	1
alcohol – history of excess	1
Post major trauma or infection	1
Therapeutic diet, e.g. already on diabetic diet	1
Feeding difficulties	
Swallowing problems, e.g. dysphagia	3
Poor appetite/altered taste	1
Poor ability to chew	1
Difficulty feeding self	1
Unwilling to eat, e.g. due to pain/anxiety	1
Weight	
Unintentional weight loss > 10% in < 3months	3

*Definition of 7 days pre- or postoperatively: if the patient's intake is poor, and surgery is planned to occur in 7 days or more, pre-operative nutritional support may be of benefit.

Case history 9.1 Nutritional assessment

A 65-year-old man is admitted to the ward with a 6-week history of diarrhoea, weight loss and poor appetite. He reported his normal weight to be 90 kg, which he knows is usually too heavy, but he has noticed his weight loss because his trousers are now too big for him. He now weighs 80 kg.

Using the nutrition checklist, the patient can be given the following score on admission:

Score	Feeding difficulties
1	Poor appetite/altered taste

Score	Weight
3	More than 10% unintentional weight loss in the last 3 months, i.e. loss of 10 kg = $\frac{10}{90}$ = 11%

The total score is 4. Therefore, either the dietitian or the doctor should be alerted; in the latter case, the doctor will then alert the dietitian.

support for those patients being admitted to hospital with existing malnutrition (Table 9.1).

Case history 9.1 illustrates the use of a nutrition checklist designed to be used on all patients within 24 h of admission. Patients are then reviewed using the checklist on a weekly basis, and the scores are recorded in nursing records. A score of ≥3 should be made apparent to the doctors and the patient referred to a dietitian.

It should be noted that:

- an overweight person can still be or become malnourished
- a patient should be weighed on admission to determine how much weight they have lost; this can also be useful for long-term monitoring of nutritional status

Fig. 9.2 illustrates appropriate nursing action for scores 1–2 in addition to a score of ≥3.

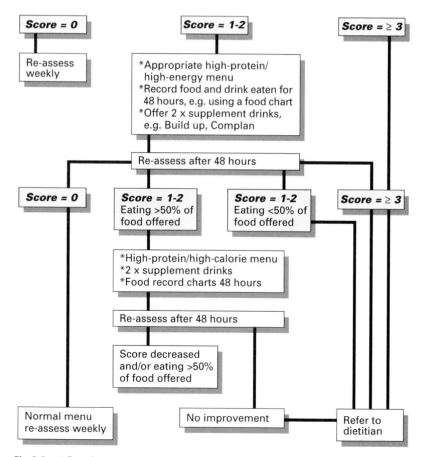

Fig 9.2   A flowchart using a nutrition checklist.

A useful phrase when considering whether to feed a patient enterally or parenterally is 'if the gut works, use it'. Benefits of enteral nutrition include maintaining the gastrointestinal structure and functional integrity, enhanced utilisation of nutrients, ease and safety of administration and lower cost.

Methods available for nutritional support

Methods range from the very simple non-invasive approach, such as encouraging a patient to eat 'little and often', to the complex high-risk invasive support involved with total parenteral nutrition (TPN).

To decide on the appropriate method to use, the first question that should be asked is 'Does the patient have a functioning gastrointestinal tract?' If the answer to this question is 'yes' then the method chosen should always be enteral feeding, i.e. use the gut. Much work has been done recently on the importance of maintaining the integrity of the gut to prevent bacterial translocation (gut origin) sepsis. Although not yet proven in human studies, it has been demonstrated that bacteria originating from the gut are able to translocate to other organs in the body to cause widespread sepsis and eventual multiple organ failure. Fig. 9.3 shows how to arrive at a decision for the most appropriate feeding method.

Food

Texture, smell and frequency of meals should be considered, e.g. soft meals presented little and often to a patient with an oesophageal stricture would be more appropriate than three large meals a day.

If the GI tract is functioning, the following should be considered:

- enteral nutrition should be encouraged, i.e. using the gastrointestinal tract
- a high-protein/high-energy menu is often used in hospitals; alternatively, the menu may highlight good choices for patients requiring extra protein and calories
- small, frequent meals, snacks and nourishing drinks if they are of the appropriate texture, e.g. of a semi-solid texture if the patient is dysphagic
- sweet or savoury supplement drinks either freshly made up on the ward, e.g. Build Up, Complan, or prepared in a carton, can or bottle, e.g. Fresubin, Entera, Ensure, Ensure Plus, Fortisip; these are best served chilled from the fridge if sweet, or warmed if savoury or flavoured
- enteral tube feeding, e.g. nasogastric, nasoduodenal, or nasojejunal tubes using special liquid products, e.g. Nutrison, Osmolite, Jevity.

On the other hand, if the GI tract is not functioning, e.g. in the case of acute pancreatitis, paralytic ileus, peritonitis, then the following nutritional support methods should be considered:

- parenteral nutrition, i.e. bypasses the gastrointestinal tract and enters the blood stream directly via a vein
  — peripheral parenteral nutrition (short-term use only)
  — central parenteral nutrition, often called total parenteral nutrition (TPN) (long-term feeding or fluid-restricted patients). For more detail, see p. 230.

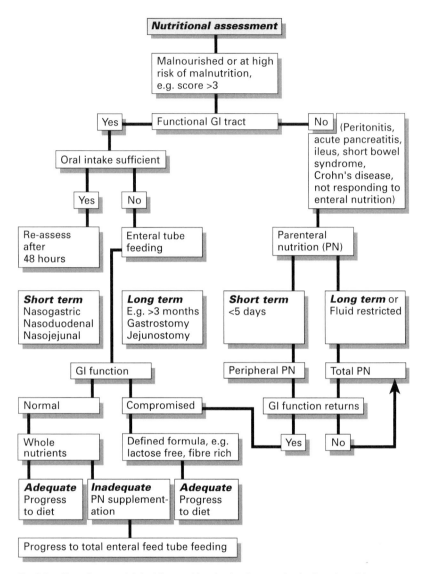

Fig 9.3 Flowchart to aid decision-making for feeding methods. (Reprinted from A.S.P.E.N. 1993. A.S.P.E.N. does not endorse this material in any form other than its entirety. For information on ordering a complete set of guidelines, contact A.S.P.E.N., 8630 Fenton Street, Suite 412, Silver Spring, MD 20910; 301\587–6315.)

Sip-feed supplements

These are either freshly made, e.g. Complan, Build Up, with milk, or ready-to-drink supplements, e.g. Ensure, Fortisip, Fresubin. Such milk-based supplements are usually nutritionally complete and should be offered in

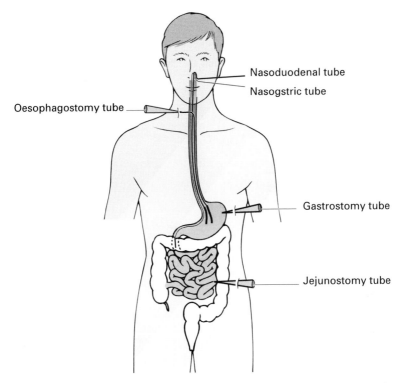

Fig 9.4 Routes for tube feeding. (Reproduced with permission from Thomas 1994).

preference to tea, coffee, squashes and clear soups, which provide few nutrients. Trials have shown that as an adjunct to normal diet, they may improve clinical outcome (Larsson et al 1990).

Tube feeding

If food and sip feeding fail to meet nutritional requirements, patients may be fed by enteral tube. There are four main routes: nasogastric, nasojejunal, gastrostomy and jejunostomy (see Fig. 9.4). Whole-protein feeds are suitable for most patients; however, if there is severe gut malfunction, e.g. Crohn's disease, then a feed in which the protein is pre-digested to peptides (peptide feed) or amino acids (elemental feed) may be indicated. Feeds are also available which are high in medium chain triglycerides (MCT), a type of fat that requires no bile salts to facilitate metabolism. A feed containing MCT could benefit any patient with steatorrhoea, such as that associated with intestinal lymphangiectasia, Crohn's disease or other established malabsorption states.

Total parenteral nutrition (TPN)

This is a final option when the gut cannot be used, e.g. for patients with acute pancreatitis or abdominal sepsis. Nutrients are infused directly into a vein. A

Table 9.2 Comparison of metabolic responses during starvation, trauma and stress

	Starvation	Trauma	Sepsis
O₂ consumption	↓	↑	↑ or ↓
Metabolic rate	↓	↑	↑ or ↓
Nitrogen loss	↑ later ↓	↑	↑↑
Gluconeogenesis, e.g.			
muscle into glucose	↑↑ later ↑	↑↑	↑↑
Ketones	↑↑	↑	↓
Energy source	Fat	Muscle and Fat	Not known

typical TPN bag will be 2.5 L in volume, with 50% of the non-protein calories coming from glucose and 50% from fat. Protein is given in the form of crystalline amino acids, and at least 1 g protein/kg body weight per day, (or 0.16 g nitrogen/kg per day) is usually provided.

Metabolic response to stress

A patient who is undergoing surgery on their GI tract or is septic due to a GI disease will show a different metabolic response compared with a patient who is simply starving. During trauma or sepsis, the loss of lean body mass and fat mass is greater than that during starvation. The body needs to provide adequate energy as glucose or ketones for the brain and other organs dependent on glucose by rapid breakdown of lean body tissue. This catabolic effect is more significant if the patient has existing malnutrition, as fuel stores, e.g. skeletal muscle and fat, may already be low (see Table 9.2).

Energy requirements

Prediction equations can be used to estimate patients' energy requirements and thus to ensure that adequate calories are being provided. The most commonly used are those by Schofield et al (1985) which calculate basal metabolic rate (BMR). The BMR is the amount of energy used to maintain life, including respiration, heartbeat and maintenance of body temperature.

For adults aged between 30 and 60 years, the equations are:

Female: BMR = 8.3 × weight (kg) + 846 kcal
Male: BMR = 11.5 × weight (kg) + 873 kcal

Once the BMR has been calculated, percentage additions are applied to account for the extra needs prompted by the disease or surgical injury. One general method for estimating the approximate energy requirements in adult patients receiving artificial nutritional support is provided by Elia (1990) (Fig. 9.5).

A combined factor for activity- and diet-induced thermogenesis (energy needed to metabolise nutrients) is also added to the BMR to give a final estimated figure of the patient's energy requirements:

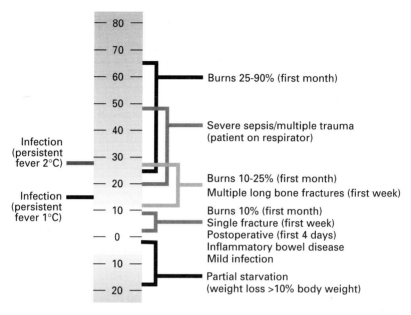

Fig 9.5 Method to estimate approximate energy requirements in an adult patient receiving artificial nutrition support. (Reproduced from Elia 1990 by kind permission of The Medicine Group (Journals) Ltd.)

Bedbound, immobile	+10% of BMR
Bedbound, mobile/sitting	+15–20%
Mobile on ward	+25%

Protein requirements, often calculated in g nitrogen/kg body weight, are also dependent on the state of the patient's metabolism, as follows:

Normal		0.17 (0.14–0.20)
Hypermetabolic	5–25%	0.20 (0.17–0.25)
	25–50%	0.25 (0.25–0.30)
	≥50%	0.30 (0.30–0.35)
If depleted		0.30 (0.20–0.40)

NB – 1 g nitrogen = 6.25 g protein

Case history 9.2 shows an example of the estimation of a patient's daily protein requirements. Based on this information, it is clear that the nutritional method for this patient should be enteral feeding, e.g. feeding with nutritionally complete sip feeds to meet requirements of approximately 2300 kcal/day and approximately 70 g protein. If the patient is unable to drink full require-

---

Case history 9.2 Estimation of protein requirement

A 32-year-old male with known Crohn's disease is admitted to hospital with a small bowel stricture. His inflammatory markers are normal and he is apyrexial. He usually weighs 70 kg, but over the last 12 weeks he has lost 7 kg in weight due to pain, nausea and anorexia to solid food. His pressure areas are intact, although he has noticed that his leg muscles have wasted slightly. Stricturoplasty surgery is highly likely during this admission unless his condition resolves medically. He is sitting out in his chair but is not yet mobile on the ward.

Nutritional assessment	Score
Muscle wasting	1
Unintentional weight loss of 10% of original body weight	3
Unwilling to eat/unable to eat properly	1
Total	5

Estimation of energy requirements		
BMR	$= 11.5 \times 63 + 873$	$= 1598$ kcal
Stress	$=$ not stressed	
Mobility and diet-induced thermogenesis	$= 20\%$	$= 320$ kcal
Increase of energy stores required	$= 400$ kcal	
Total	$= 2318$ kcal/day	

Estimation of protein requirements
63 kg $\times$ 0.17 $= 11$g N/day or 69 g protein/day

Does the patient have a functioning GI tract? Yes, although tolerance to solids is poor.

---

ments orally, a fine-bore nasogastric tube could be suitable for short-term feeding and a standard whole-protein enteral feed could be used to ensure that requirements are met, e.g. overnight nasogastric feeding.

Not only do particular diseases of the GI tract have an adverse effect on a patient's nutritional status but diet also has an important role in the management of certain diseases.

THERAPEUTIC DIETS FOR DISEASES OF THE GASTROINTESTINAL TRACT

Oesophagus

Any disease which causes a narrowing of the oesophageal lumen or a reduction in the elasticity of its walls will interfere with the delivery of food from the mouth to the stomach. Inevitably, malnutrition results.

Nutritional consequences of dysphagia

In both benign strictures and malignant tumours of the oesophagus, difficulty in swallowing solid foods may progress to dysphagia with semi-solids and later with liquids. Pain and anxiety associated with eating or inappropriate food choice mean that patients usually present with weight loss. As with all patients in whom malnutrition is suspected, an assessment should be made of the extent of malnutrition. If dysphagia is severe, a patient may also be dehydrated. Rehydration and nutritional support prior to treatment are often necessary.

Nutritional management of dysphagia

Dysphagia with solids
- A semi-solid diet is required.
- Small meals should be given often.
- Effervescent fluids are helpful.
- Extra sauce or gravy will facilitate swallowing.
- Consider the use of liquid or semi-solid nutritional supplements.

Dysphagia with semi-solids
- A puréed or liquidised diet is required.
- The addition of liquids is necessary to achieve the correct texture; use soup, milk or white sauce rather than low-calorie fluids such as water.
- Add extra milk, butter or cheese to potatoes and other liquidised vegetables to improve energy and protein intake.
- Foods should look, smell and taste good.
- Encourage milk-based drinks, e.g. milkshakes and milky coffee, rather than low-energy fluids, e.g. squash, tea, water.
- A liquid supplement is likely to be essential.

Dysphagia with liquidised food
- A fluid diet is needed.
- Nutritional supplements that are complete in their composition will be needed.
- Fluids can be sipped or taken via a nasogastric feeding tube.

Dysphagia with liquid
- Initially, the patient should be rehydrated with fluids intravenously.
- A fine-bore tube should be passed, if possible, for enteral nutritional support.
- Consider the placement of a gastrostomy feeding tube if intubation is not possible or if dysphagia to liquids is likely to be long-term.
- Consider total parenteral nutrition prior to treatment if intubation is not possible, or if gastrostomy is unsuitable and the patient's diagnosis indicates it.

Nutritional consequences of the treatment of dysphagia
Certain treatments of dysphagia may also have nutritional consequences, requiring careful management

Surgical treatment (see also nutritional consequences and management following gastric surgery).
- The integrity of the anastomosis needs confirmation before feeding.

- Peripheral nutrition, TPN or jejunostomy feeding will be needed postoperatively if the patient is malnourished pre-operatively.
- Gradual progression from oral fluids to light diet should be implemented with associated phasing out of TPN of jejunostomy feed.

Radiotherapy
- This may make dysphagia temporarily worse due to tissue inflammation and swelling.
- Nasogastric feeding should be considered if the oral intake is insufficient.
- Continuation of a soft semi-solid diet is likely to be possible.
- Nutritional supplements should be considered.

Insertion of a Celestin or Atkinson tube
- Meals should be small, frequent and chewed well.
- Textures may still need to be modified.
- New bread should be avoided. Day-old bread and crispbreads are usually better tolerated.
- Nutritional supplements, e.g. Build Up, Fortisip, should be used.
- After eating a meal, a small volume of fizzy drink, e.g. lemonade, should be sipped to help clear the tube of food particles.

Stomach
The stomach functions as a reservoir for food, and secretes acid and pepsin to facilitate digestion. Diseases of the stomach and surgical intevention will have profound effects on gastric function and therefore nutritional intake.

Nutritional consequences of cancer of the stomach
Anorexia, nausea, vomiting, pain on eating and the actual disease process itself can all result in loss of lean body tissue and fat. Gastric surgery will disrupt the various mechanisms regulating the correct functioning of the gastrointestinal tract, and will often lead to a number of problems (Table 9.3).

Small intestine
The small intestine is the main site of absorption of nutrients. Disease of the small bowel and surgical intervention are highly likely to cause some degree of malabsorption for one or more nutrients (Fig. 9.6). The result of such malabsorption will interfere with a patient's nutritional status.

The aims of nutritional management are:

- dietary treatment of the primary disorder, e.g. the exclusion of gluten in coeliac disease
- daily replacement of lost fluids and electrolytes
- restoration of optimum nutritional state.

Coeliac disease
In coeliac disease, gluten damages the lining of the small intestine so that food cannot be absorbed effectively. Gluten is a protein found in wheat, rye, barley and possibly oats. The possible nutritional consequences of coeliac disease are:

Table 9.3 Potential problems following gastric surgery and their nutritional management

Problem	Dietary management
Early satiety	Small frequent meals. Fluids should be taken 1 h before or after meals. Food should be chewed well
Fear of eating	Encouragement. Relaxation before and after meals. Avoid large meals
Reflux	Avoidance of strong coffee, alcohol, spicy foods, chocolate, citrus fruits, fatty foods. Avoid eating late in the evening. Avoid smoking
Early dumping syndrome	Avoid sugary foods and drinks. Take liquids before or after meals. Encourage protein and fat-rich meals. Avoid alcohol
Diarrhoea	Management is for early dumping together with antidiarrhoeal drugs (codeine and loperamide)
Bile vomiting	No dietary management. Drugs to accelerate gastric emptying may help
Late dumping syndrome	If acute attack, give glucose or sugar by mouth. For prevention of late dumping, see early dumping
Malabsorption of fat	Reduction in fat intake. Replacement of calories with a glucose polymer or medium chain triglycerides
Malabsorption of calcium	Give calcium and vitamin D supplement
Iron	Give oral iron
Folate	Give oral folate
Vitamin B_{12}	Consider intramuscular B_{12} injections every 3 months

- diarrhoea
- pain
- weight loss
- anaemia
- lethargy
- nausea.

Diet therapy

- A lifetime elimination of all gluten from the diet is essential following which 85% of adults and all children will make a full recovery, which will be sustained as long as gluten is not reintroduced.

- Advice and counselling on a gluten-free diet should be provided by an experienced dietitian. This diet should integrate fully into the patient's lifestyle.

- Patients should be encouraged to belong to the Coeliac Society, which aims to promote the welfare of adults and children who have been medically

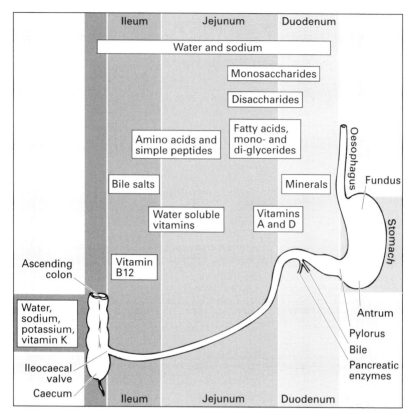

Fig 9.6   Sites for absorption of nutrients in the gastrointestinal tract. (Reproduced with permission from Thomas 1994).

diagnosed as having coeliac disease or dermatitis herpetiformis. Those on their mailing list receive a list of gluten-free manufactured products (the 'food list'). This list is updated every year and is published in April.

• Gluten-free flour, bread, biscuits, pasta and other specialised dietary products are available to coeliacs. Such products provide bulk, variety and essential nutrients to ensure an adequate energy intake. Several of these products, e.g. bread, pasta, flour and some biscuits, are available on prescription for patients diagnosed with coeliac disease.

• The gluten-free diet must be balanced with respect to all other nutrients. Generally there is no need for restriction on milk and dairy produce, eggs, fish, meat, fruit, vegetables, rice or corn.

Unexplained weight loss, anaemia with folate deficiency, and diarrhoea or biopsy showing continued villous atrophy may be signs of gluten ingestion. Referral to a dietitian for a detailed dietary reassessment is recommended in these cases.

Crohn's disease

If the Crohn's disease is severe and the small bowel is affected, the likelihood of nutritional deficiencies is high. Weight loss occurs in 65–75% of patients with Crohn's (Fleming 1994). Common deficiencies include energy, protein, iron, folic acid and vitamin B_{12}. Sodium and fluid depletion are also prevalent in patients with persistent diarrhoea, and zinc, magnesium and other trace element deficiencies may occur.

The reasons for these deficiencies include:

- poor food intake due to pain, nausea, fear of eating, anorexia, malaise and imposition of restricted diets
- malabsorption due to decreased effective absorption area, bile acid deficiency leading to fat and fat-soluble vitamin malabsorption, bacteria overgrowth, rapid transit time and drug–nutrient interaction
- blood electrolyte, protein, mineral and trace element loss due to active inflammation
- hypercatabolism from infection, inflammation and fever
- long-term use of corticosteroids, which may cause a prolonged state of catabolism with tissue breakdown, negative nitrogen balance, impaired wound healing, decreased resistance to infection, increased capillary fragility and osteoporosis
- the catabolic effects of surgery with possible short bowel syndrome, B_{12} deficiency (terminal ileum resection) and fat malabsorption.

The aims of any dietary treatment for Crohn's disease must be to improve and/or maintain a satisfactory nutritional status during both active disease and remission.

Diet therapies

'Normal' diet. For most people in remission, emphasis should be placed on the known positive benefits of a well-balanced diet, rather than on the less certain benefits of dietary restrictions. Most will be able to eat a normal varied diet, perhaps having to avoid certain food excesses or specific foods which can also upset people that are in good health.

Any diet restriction should only be made on medical advice.

Low-fibre (low non-starch polysaccharide) diet. A low-fibre diet may be useful in Crohn's patients who have a stricture or history of obstruction. The diet should therefore be low in wholegrain cereals, nuts, fruit and vegetables. Nutrient intake of vitamin C and folic acid will therefore be reduced and so suitable alternatives must be found or an appropriate vitamin supplement prescribed.

High-fibre (high non-starch polysaccharide) diet. Heaton et al (1979) studied the effects of a high-fibre, low-refined-sugar diet in 32 patients with Crohn's disease, and found that they had significantly fewer and shorter admissions to hospital than did a group of matched controls. This was a small study and subsequent studies have shown no significant difference in clinical course between patients treated with a high-fibre diet and controls (Ritchie et al 1987).

Patients with stricturing or narrowing should be advised against a high-fibre diet.

Low-fat diet. Malabsorption of fat in Crohn's disease may occur after resection of the terminal ileum or as a result of bacterial overgrowth. Steatorrhoea will also lead to losses of calcium, magnesium and possibly zinc. Fat restriction may be useful in proven cases of steatorrhoea, although it should be remembered that fat is an excellent source of energy, providing 9 kcal/g (37.8 kJ/g), and must be replaced with either carbohydrate or medium chain triglyceride (MCT) supplements. MCT supplements will be absorbed as they do not require bile salts for emulsification. MCT supplements include oils for frying or for use in baking and as milk substitutes. MCT must be introduced into the diet gradually because it can cause an osmotic diarrhoea. The diet may need to be supplemented with fat-soluble vitamins (A, D, E and K), calcium and essential fatty acids if it is strict.

Low-lactose diet. Functional and structural damage to the jejunal mucosa may result in hypolactasia, although conflicting reports exist about the prevalence and its importance (Park et al 1990, Pironi et al 1988). However, despite hypolactasia, most studies suggest that small quantities of lactose, equivalent to less than 240 ml milk/day, are tolerated (Suarez et al 1995). Unless supervised, a reduction in milk and dairy products can lead to deficits in calcium, protein and energy. Hypolactasia should be specifically diagnosed by means of a lactose tolerance breath test.

Total parenteral nutrition (primary therapy). TPN was initially used in Crohn's disease if patients were malnourished. Observation of improvement not only in nutritional intake but also in disease activity led to the proposal of using TPN as a primary treatment. It was thought that bowel rest was the mechanism for inducing remission, but a study by Greenburg et al (1988) cast doubt on this theory. They found no significant difference in outcome between those on TPN and nil by mouth, and those being enterally fed.

Total enteral nutrition (primary therapy). Enteral or TPN are likely to facilitate remission in 60–80% of patients with acute exacerbation of Crohn's disease, although the mechanisms whereby nutrition reduces disease activity are poorly understood, controversial and require further research. Several mechanisms have been proposed to explain the apparent therapeutic action of enteral nutrition, including bowel rest (although this is doubtful; see Greenburg et al 1988); reduction of the antigenic load on the gut; decreasing permeability changes and protein loss from the inflamed gut; decreasing faecal bile salts; actively nourishing the bowel and improving the nutritional status of the patient.

Current evidence points to enteral feeding, rather than TPN, as being the preferred method of nutritional support to treat active Crohn's disease, particularly among children and adolescents, except when use of the gastrointestinal tract is not possible, e.g. in the early stages of short bowel syndrome, high-grade bowel obstruction or in the presence of high output fistulae.

Initially amino acid-based feeds known as elemental diets were used. These were first shown to be as effective as steroids in achieving short-term remission (O'Morain et al 1984). Later studies found peptide, or semi-elemental diets and even whole-protein or polymeric feeds to be equally effective in most cases, i.e. a non-elemental diet is as effective as an elemental one. The main advantages non-elemental diets have are that they cost less and are more palatable. However, the usefulness of any formulated food as the sole primary therapy in active Crohn's remains controversial. In a meta-analysis of enteral nutrition as a primary treatment of active Crohn's disease, it was concluded that corticosteroids are more effective than enteral nutrition (Griffiths et al 1995). Enteral nutrition is still of therapeutic benefit, however, even if the efficacy does not equal that of steroid treatment. There are also risk/benefit considerations of enteral nutrition over steroids in children or adolescents, due to the known linear growth stunting effects of steroids. Enteral nutrition, either by sip feeding or tube feeding, has been found to be useful as a means of supplementing the nutrition of depleted Crohn's patients in remission.

Short bowel syndrome

Short bowel syndrome refers to the clinical effects of the removal of a large portion of the small intestine. It is characterised by malnutrition secondary to diarrhoea, fluid and electrolyte disturbances and malabsorption (Allard & Jeejeebhoy 1989). Conditions which can result in short bowel syndrome include mesenteric infarction, Crohn's disease, radiation enteritis, trauma, bowel tumours, necrotising enterocolitis and intestinal atresia in infants.

Nutrient absorption occurs throughout the small bowel. When the jejunum is removed, the ileum takes over most of the lost function. Although a loss of even 100 cm of terminal ileum may cause steatorrhoea, removal of up to 33% of the small bowel results in no malnutrition, and removal of up to 50% can usually be tolerated without TPN support. Patients with resections of more than 75%, however, usually require TPN to avoid dehydration and/or malnutrition. Some patients may need TPN at home for survival. Nutritional deficiencies will depend on the extent and location of the small bowel resection. A summary of the progressive management of patients with short bowel syndrome is provided in Box 9.1.

Patients with short bowel syndrome, where the colon is intact, have an increased risk of urinary oxalate stones. This is because fat malabsorption causes calcium and magnesium soaps to form, decreasing free ion availability. Oxalate absorption is increased because these ions usually bind with oxalate to form insoluble, poorly absorbed oxalate salts.

Patients with steatorrhoea and an intact colon should be advised to limit foods high in oxalates, such as chocolate, tea, squash, rhubarb, tomatoes and strawberries. Fat intake should be reduced to tolerance, perhaps with the use of MCT supplements to increase the energy intake. Calcium supplements should be given. A happy medium needs to be found between a dietary fat intake that maintains good nutrition and a restriction of fat to reduce steatorrhoea.

Box 9.1 Summary of the progressive management of patients with a short small intestine and large loses (Lennard-Jones & Wood 1991)

Phase 1: gaining stability and assessing basal intestinal output
- Patient should sip fluid by mouth
- Intravenous replacement
  - initial requirement should be judged from clinical and biochemical evidence of dehydration. Fluids used should be mainly normal saline, as sodium deficiency is the major problem. During the first 24 h, 3 L of saline may be needed in addition to the maintenance volume if there is prerenal uraemia or hypotension
- Intravenous maintenance
  - water: previous day's losses + 1L should be given
  - sodium: previous day's losses judged as 100 mmol/L of effluent + 80 mmol should be given
  - potassium: 80 mmol/day should be given
  - magnesium: 8–14 mmol/day should be given
  - nutrients: these should be given only if there is severe malnutrition and it seems unlikely that enteral replacement will succeed

Phase 2: gradual transfer to oral fluids and nutrients
- Continue intravenous replacement so that there is no pressure to eat or drink
- Make additions one at a time and assess effect on intestinal output
  - start oral fluids (500 ml/day)
  - start food but discourage drinks with meals
  - start sipping glucose-electrolyte solution up to 1L daily
  - start magnesium oxide

(12 mmol/daily) if serum magnesium is low
  - start antidiarrhoeal drugs such as loperamide (2 or 4 mg up to four times daily) (the syrup may be preferable in patients with rapid transit, or the capsules may be opened) and/or codeine phosphate (30 mg up to four times daily). These drugs should be given 30–60 min before meals
  - start a gastric antisecretory drug if intestinal output is very high

Phase 3: complete transfer to enteral feeding if possible
- Encourage snacks
- Consider the need for nasogastric feeds
- If it is impossible to maintain electrolyte balance or nutrition by the oral route, start training the patient to self-administer intravenous supplements

Phase 4: rehabilitation
- A seriously malnourished patient needs to regain strength before being able to care for him- or herself. If home enteral tube feeding or parenteral feeding is necessary, training can be started only when the patient is able to cope with it.
  Explanation to the patient's family and employer, and possibly modifications to the home or job, may be needed before a patient can undertake full activity

Phase 5: long-term care
- When the patient returns home regular supervision is needed. It may be possible to stop tube or intravenous supplements once malnutrition is corrected and intestinal adaptation has occurred

Large intestine

Ulcerative colitis

The incidence of nutritional deficiencies in ulcerative colitis (UC) is not as common as in Crohn's disease. Weight loss has been said to occur in 18–62% of patients with the disease (Fleming 1994). If weight loss is seen, it is during an acute attack which usually results in inadequate energy intake because of anorexia, pain, vomiting and diarrhoea. If diarrhoea is profuse, fluid and electrolyte depletion may result. Anaemia may also occur due to chronic blood loss from an inflamed colonic mucosa.

There is no evidence to suggest that nutrition has a primary therapeutic effect on patients with UC. However, nutrition support or diet therapy may improve a patient's nutritional status if malnourished, or may prevent at-risk patients from developing specific deficiencies. With UC, there is no malabsorption of nutrients in the small bowel, but other reasons for nutrient deficiencies are the same as for Crohn's disease.

Diet therapies (adjuvant therapies)

'Normal' diet. In remission, a normal balanced diet is recommended. Avoidance of foods for symptom management is individual and often not required.

Low-fibre (low non-starch polysaccharide) diet. A low-fibre diet may be advised during mild or moderate attacks of UC. If diet remains restricted in this way, the intake of vitamins and minerals should be assessed.

High-fibre (high non-starch polysaccharide) diet. This may be advised in those with distal colonic or rectal disease who have difficulty passing hard faeces. A high-fibre diet should also accompany a higher fluid intake – at least eight cups of fluid a day.

Low-fat diet. Low fat diets do not appear to be useful in UC.

Low-lactose diet. In UC, hypolactasia can occur during acute attacks, although this usually improves when patients go into remission. Specific diagnosis is advised, as for Crohn's disease, and a degree of tolerance to lactose may still exist, i.e. 240 ml milk a day despite hypolactasia (Suarez et al 1995).

Total parenteral nutrition. TPN does not influence disease activity in patients with severe acute exacerbations of UC. TPN may, however, benefit those patients already identified as being malnourished, in which surgery is being considered and where the enteral route is not possible.

Total enteral nutrition. During a severe attack, therapy may include taking nothing orally for 5–7 days. However, some clinicians will allow enteral sip feeds or even a light diet during this period without affecting the clinical outcome. As for any gastrointestinal condition, enteral feeding (sipping orally or tube) will benefit a patient, if malnourished in the remission phase, as an adjuvant therapy.

Colorectal cancer

Patients often present with weight loss and malnutrition. Pre-operative nutrition, as well as postoperative nutritional support, is therefore important. The enteral route should be the first choice – either an oral diet plus supplements or tube feeding will help to meet the patient's nutritional requirements. Overnight nasogastric feeding is a useful means of topping up energy and protein levels without intefering with dietary intake during the day.

Following resection, some patients may require a temporary or permanent ileostomy or colostomy. They should be encouraged to have as normal a diet as possible, but to avoid any foods which cause the stool consistency or odour to be unacceptable to them. High-fibre foods such as wholegrain bread, fruit and vegetables should not be discouraged as a good fibre intake ensures efficient functioning of the stoma.

Patients with ileostomies usually lose both electrolytes (sodium and potassium) and fluid, which necessitates an increase of these nutrients for at least 6–8 weeks. After this time, the ileum adapts and the usual diet will suffice. Adding a little extra salt to food and choosing foods that are rich in potassium, such as bananas, potatoes, coffee and orange juice, will help to boost electrolyte intakes in the initial postoperative phase.

TOTAL PARENTERAL NUTRITION

What is TPN?

The human dietary components are energy, protein, vitamins, minerals and water. Patients unable to eat still need these components and they may be delivered in a liquid form via a central venous catheter into the heart. This is known as total parenteral nutrition, or TPN.

Energy

The main sources of energy are carbohydrate and fat, but protein also provides a useful contribution.

Carbohydrate

Glucose is the carbohydrate of choice for patients receiving TPN since high calorific doses may be given without causing venous damage.

Fat

Fat is another important energy source for the TPN patient. The combination of fat and carbohydrate provides a balanced calorific input without the risk of complications associated with TPN regimens using glucose alone.

Protein

Unfortunately, the body does not have an unlimited protein store – skeletal muscle is the main reserve of protein during starvation. It can be seen, for example, how the loss of skeletal muscle makes a patient very weak, tissue slow to heal and immune responses sluggish.

Protein is composed of two separate groups of amino acids – *essential*, which the body is unable to synthesise, and *non-essential*. The body depends on the presence of both types of amino acids to meet nitrogen requirements.

A fit and normal adult will have a good or equal nitrogen balance, i.e. the nitrogen retained from the diet will equal the nitrogen lost from the body. Additional nitrogen is excreted. In nitrogen-deficient patients, skeletal muscle is broken down to supply amino acids unless enteral or parenteral feeding is commenced to provide an alternative source. Nitrogen that is broken down from protein is largely excreted as urea, which is why 24-hourly urine collections help to estimate the loss of nitrogen. This will be discussed later in this chapter.

Vitamins and minerals
The major minerals – sodium, potassium, calcium, magnesium and phosphate – are all required in relatively large amounts, which vary from patient to patient. Vitamins and the remaining minerals are required only in very small quantities but are vital to their interaction with enzymes.

Water
Water is an essential daily diet component. Artificial feeding will increase fluid or water requirements, as additional urine will be produced to aid in the excretion of waste products.

SELECTION OF CANDIDATES FOR TPN

The decision to provide a patient with nutritional support must be based on an informed assessment of the patient's condition. Audit demonstrates that the need and indications for TPN are increasing annually, consistent with the rise in the number of patients receiving TPN at home (currently about 300 in the UK).

The method of providing nutrition is determined very simply by the question: 'Is the gastrointestinal tract functional?' If the gut is functioning, enteral nutrition is obviously the method of choice; if not, parenteral nutrition should be instituted (see Fig. 9.7).

Prior to any form of nutritional support being implemented, it is very important that the patient's nutritional status is assessed accurately by the nutritional support team (NST). Nutritional assessment is based upon the patient's history, the disease process and the effect both factors have on the patient's body weight.

The relevance of TPN in gastroenterology
Gastroenterology patients who may require TPN fall into three definite groups.

Group I
The first group of patients suffer from functional bowel failure. This may be due to any of the following:

- bowel surgery
- malignancy of the small bowel

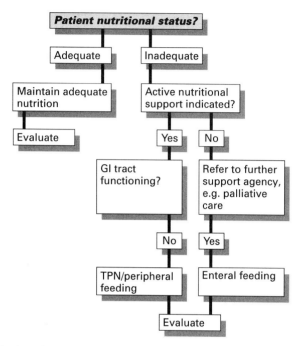

Fig 9.7 Selection of candidates for TPN.

- malignancy of the upper gastrointestinal tract
- Crohn's disease (IBD)
- pancreatitis and pseudocysts
- malabsorption, i.e. coeliac disease
- intestinal obstruction
- oesophageal surgery.

Although bowel surgery may include a split ileostomy, permitting the bowel to rest, TPN can be used as a form of medical defunctioning of the colon, in order to avoid the complications and risks of surgery for patients with extensive colonic Crohn's disease. Abdominal pain, partial intestinal obstruction, poor appetite and nausea mean that these patients often present in a poorly nourished state. Constant abdominal pain can mean that a patient is unable to tolerate any oral intake, or indeed have any interest in food at all, and TPN can therefore be of great benefit in providing essential nourishment.

TPN provides a comprehensive nutritional regimen which prevents the starvation that might otherwise occur in some of the patients in this group. The treatment of the underlying disease is paramount in overcoming nutritional problems, but TPN may be instrumental in correcting specific nutritional defects.

The opportunity for established centres to provide home TPN has revolutionised the future for many patients with gastrointestinal problems and for those who have less than 70 cm of small bowel. The latter group will need home TPN on an indefinite basis. They may suffer from radiation enteritis, major gut resection due to vascular embolisation or congenital gut absorption problems.

Group 2

The second group suffer from bowel incompetence which may be due to any of the following:

- acute surgical episodes involving gut resection with anastomosis
- overwhelming sepsis, resulting in gut stasis
- burns affecting the gut, e.g. radiation enteritis, chemical burns
- internal or external fistulae
- congenital gut disorders requiring surgical intervention.

This group of patients will require nutritional support for at the least several days and often for a number of weeks.

The majority of complications following bowel resection and anastomosis are related to anastomotic leaks and wound healing, involving wound infections, which can be attributed to some extent to malnutrition (Buzby et al 1988).

If, during surgery, a clinical decision is made to give parenteral feeding, a central venous feeding line may be inserted at the time for this purpose.

Postoperatively, the gut function will be impaired and the mucosa is less able to absorb fluid or nutrients. For many patients undergoing emergency surgery for excessive bleeding or intra-abdominal sepsis, pre-operative nutritional support will not have been considered.

TPN given over a period of less than 4 days will have no significant or measurable effect on the patient's nutritional state. A period of 5–7 days is considered the minimum to produce beneficial effects.

Group 3

The third group of patients who may require TPN suffer from a loss of bowel function due to any of the following:

- massive resection due to infarction, as a result of mesenteric thrombosis
- advanced Crohn's disease
- malignancy
- bowel obstruction due to adhesions, malignancy or fibrosis
- enterocutaneous fistulae due to Crohn's disease, malignancy or previous surgery.

In any of these situations, major resection of the gut may be necessary. When more than 50% of the bowel is resected, absorptive impairment tends to be long-term or permanent, in spite of the reserve and intestinal adaptation. The ileum has a particularly important role in the absorption of vitamin B_{12} and bile salts – resection will disrupt this process.

When resection exceeds 75% of the bowel, the patient's nutritional status cannot be maintained without support in the form of TPN, which must be instituted promptly to avoid malnutrition. Every effort must still be made to introduce oral feeding where possible. Many patients may still be able to enjoy the social aspect of eating, despite being unable to absorb enteral nutrients, and yet be successfully supported by parenteral nutrition.

Patients who have small bowel resection plus severe diarrhoea have an increased requirement for zinc – up to 12–15 mg per day. In addition, the urine output can be up to 1 L/day. These fluid losses may be difficult to monitor accurately, which is why regular biochemical assessment is essential when using parenteral nutrition in this type of patient.

Patients who have enterocutaneous fistulae suffer substantial fluid losses and require accurate measurements of fluid and electrolyte balances. Patients with excessive fistula output must be regularly monitored for the status of their trace elements of zinc, chromium, selenium and magnesium.

TPN may be required long-term until the fistula heals naturally or is surgically resected. In the early stages of the fistula healing process, enteral fluids must be avoided in order to allow every opportunity for healing to take place. Whether the healing is natural or by surgical resection, enteral nutrition must be introduced slowly alongside TPN until a stage is reached when the patient can tolerate 1000 kcal by mouth, when TPN can then be reduced or stopped. In very long-term cases, i.e. awaiting fistulae to heal, home TPN may be necessary.

The length of time a patient receives TPN during fistula management depends on the underlying gastroenterological pathology and the type of fistula concerned. Even so, fistula healing hardly ever replaces sound surgical principles, which may eventually be necessary. It must be borne in mind that some fistulae never heal (Fazio et al 1985).

Selection of patients for home TPN (HPN)

These patients are generally limited to those with non-malignant diseases, massive gut resection due to infarction, Crohn's disease, enterocutaneous fistulae or congenital gut absorptive diseases. TPN is the one and only advisable type of nutrition for them. Some may require TPN for the rest of their lives, or indefinitely, in order to supplement their dietary and fluid intake.

These patients usually administer TPN overnight so that they may continue to work or attend school with the minimum of disruption to their personal routine. Patient selection is the key factor to successful HPN; living conditions are a secondary consideration.

A structured training period using the local TPN protocol is vital for patients requiring HPN. Experienced gastroenterology nurses will be able to design a detailed teaching programme which stresses the importance of simplicity and safety. Consistency in teaching and communication is another important issue. The gastroenterology nursing team or clinical nurse specialist/TPN should allow at least 2–3 weeks to carry out this detailed training and assessment of the patient's living conditions.

The financial implications for a patient receiving HPN over long periods, or indeed for life, are high, around £3000–4000/month (1996 prices).

Successful HPN depends entirely on the patient's or the carer's ability to provide detailed daily care and attention. Not all patients will be capable of performing the tasks associated with HPN, due to other medical problems or the tremor some patients develop while receiving this method of nutrition. The social circumstances of some patients may not allow for carers to be available to provide the detailed care necessary for HPN.

Appropriate patient selection is therefore imperative for the safe administration of TPN in the community, enhancing the patient's quality of life and therefore justifying a huge financial outlay. Case history 9.3 illustrates the problems that may be encountered in patients requiring HPN.

Following a directive from the Department of Health in April 1995, each district health authority has a choice as to who provides the service for TPN – the local hospital or an external pharmaceutical company. In either case, the cost of providing nutrition of this type, although entirely worthwhile, is extremely high. The nutritional support team can be instrumental in reducing costs and avoiding confusion by standardising the equipment a patient of this type will need when at home on TPN.

A support network for HPN patients is essential, preferably using a named gastroenterology nurse or ward in the case of emergency. Patients must be made aware of the complications that can occur while they are receiving TPN and know how to resolve them or who to gain assistance from, day or night.

Stability of biochemistry and haematology is obviously essential before a home TPN patient can be discharged and the frequency of monitoring reduced to once a week. Home patients should be seen initially at monthly intervals by the consultant in charge of the case, who should have an interest and understanding of TPN. If stability is maintained, follow-up visits can be reduced to once every 3 months. The gastroenterology nursing team should be available on these occasions if the patient should require support or advice on issues other than TPN.

Monitoring of home patients is very important. Many patients will require little or no adjustment to their nutritional requirements, except in the case of paediatric patients where regular adjustments will be necessary in order for their growth to be maintained. Some patients will notice a steady weight gain, particularly those who are able to tolerate enteral nutrition in small quantities. Regular monitoring by the gastroenterology team will ensure excessive weight gain or loss will not occur.

It is not uncommon for lipid levels to rise in patients who have been on home TPN for long periods. Reduction of calorie intake in the form of lipids may be necessary, a decision the medical team and the dietitian specialising in gastroenterology will take at the outpatients' clinic.

The central line itself requires careful assessment at these reviews. Thrombosis and blockage can present in the long-term use of central venous catheters, which can be avoided if the patient is monitored effectively by an experienced team familiar with the use of these catheters.

Case history 9.3 Assessment for HPN

Mrs Jones, married with six children, required a laparotomy due to spontaneous massive infarction of her small bowel. Intestinal resection was necessary, leaving 70 cm of jejunum. Mrs Jones developed overwhelming sepsis and suffered a cardiac arrest due to ventricular tachycardia. Long-term positive pressure ventilation was needed and she required a tracheostomy.

The problems Mrs Jones presented with on referral for HPN were as follows:

• severe weakness, e.g. unable to wash or brush her hair
• inability to communicate due to tracheostomy
• low morale
• pain
• infection
• malnutrition due to excessive output from jejunostomy and general hypercatabolic state
• poor venous access.

Following such an extensive resection of the bowel, it was clear that Mrs Jones would require permanent nutritional support in the form of TPN.

A careful and detailed history was obtained from Mrs Jones and her husband. Baseline measurements of weight, biochemistry, haematology, vitamin and trace elements and anthropmetry were recorded. Due to Mrs Jones' frustration at not being able to communicate, plus her weakness and low spirits, it was decided to delay HPN education. However, discharge arrangements were considered early and communication was set up with her GP and district nurse. In the absence of formal teaching, the principles and reasons for associating fluid intake and output were discussed with both Mr and Mrs Jones. A routine began to develop, with the nursing team weighing Mrs Jones at a similar time each day, establishing a procedure that would be helpful on her eventual discharge.

At this stage, a visit to Mrs Jones' home was arranged by the gastroenterology nursing team, to assess whether living conditions were conducive for HPN. The family home proved to be eminently suitable, with a bedroom containing a wash basin, ideal for the preparation and connection of a patient to TPN.

Due to Mrs Jones' severely malnourished state, it was no surprise to find that most of the results of her investigations were abnormal, particularly her serum selenium which was 0.01 (normal = 0.8–1.6 μmol/L). Selenium is a trace element involved in protecting the body against free radical damage. In Mrs Jones' case, selenium levels were very low and this undoubtedly contributed to her severe muscle weakness. In addition to her nutritional requirements, 1.2 μmol/L of sodium selenite was added daily to her TPN. Slowly the muscle strength in her limbs and chest wall improved and she was able to cough effectively; she began mobilising slowly with the help of the physiotherapists and the nursing team.

Mrs Jones' nutritional requirements stabilised once her infections were controlled and she developed equal nitrogen balance, with only electrolyte alterations proving necessary occasionally if stoma losses exceeded her norm.

Mrs Jones' tracheostomy had been in position for many weeks and an

---

Case history 9.3 *(cont'd)*

---

established tract had formed. The tube was removed and dressed, encouraging the incision to heal, and within a few days Mrs Jones was able to whisper a few words.

Mrs Jones had always appeared to be a diffident lady, preferring her own company. Despite the privacy of her own room, concentration continued to pose a problem due to the levels of analgesia and night sedation she required. Once these were reviewed, Mrs Jones' concentration span improved and brief teaching sessions were possible.

The stomatherapist became involved, gently directing Mrs Jones in the changing of her jejunostomy bag and advising her on the importance of caring for the skin around the stoma site.

One month following admission, Mrs Jones was able to begin learning the aspects of care associated with home TPN. These sessions were very short but gave the gastroenterology nursing team time to build a close relationship with Mrs Jones and her family. Slowly, her confidence grew and the teaching sessions lengthened as her powers of concentration also grew.

Venous access continued to be a problem and it was decided to insert a double lumen Hickman line for when Mrs Jones went home. This type of line is made of silicone, is strong and is often used for long periods of intravenous therapy in the community.

At this stage, Mrs Jones' medical team decided to introduce a light enteral diet plus oral fluids. Initially, the output from the jejunostomy was excessive, but minor adjustments to her diet eventually resulted in manageable losses, e.g. <700 ml daily. Once her nutritional state was stabilised, Mrs Jones received TPN overnight, mobility became less of a problem and she was able to join her family on short outings in the car. The nursing team encouraged Mrs Jones to dress and develop a routine for her eventual discharge. This added to her increasing confidence.

At this stage, Mrs Jones was receiving the occasional night sedation and rarely required analgesia.

Eleven weeks following her admission, Mrs Jones had learned the advanced principles of the aseptic technique associated with home TPN and was competent in every aspect of this and her stoma care. With the support network in position, she went home.

Unfortunately, 4 weeks later, blood results demonstrated an increase in WBC to 18 mmol/L, together with a sudden rise and fall in temperature. Mrs Jones was admitted as an emergency and was found to be dehydrated, febrile and very anxious. Blood cultures grew *Staphylococcus epidermidis*. A diagnosis of central line sepsis was made. The microbiologists advised that the line should be removed, due to the extent of infection; i.v. vancomycin was commenced. Peripheral fluids were given for 5 days. A new Hickman line was inserted 5 days later and aseptic principles reinforced.

Mrs Jones began to gain weight and the dietitian advised her further on suitable food types for patients with a jejunostomy. Vitamin and trace element assays were repeated and found to be within normal limits. The episode of central line sepsis proved to be a salutary lesson and an experience she did not wish to repeat.

After this one infection of the central line, Mrs Jones began to enjoy normal family life and suffered no further complications.

NURSING CARE IN TPN

Any patient receiving TPN will require precise and meticulous monitoring and nursing care. Problems associated with i.v. nutrition are likely to be complex (Table 9.4), the management of TPN being only one aspect of the patient's care.

Daily observations need to be assessed by the nursing staff and include the following areas.

Accurate fluid balance

Reliable fluid balance will indicate to the gastroenterology team precise losses from fistulae or stomas. Nitrogen excretion and balance can only be assessed accurately when such losses are collected, measured and recorded. With this information the nutritional support team (NST) will be able to respond to changes in the patient's nutritional requirements. A malnourished patient, due to a low serum albumin, may be unable to tolerate large fluid volumes and may demonstrate this in the form of ankle and sacral oedema. It is equally important for the gastroenterology team and NST to recognise the early signs of dehydration by considering the patient's insensible losses and correcting the balance accordingly.

Urine testing

This should be performed prior to a patient commencing TPN and thereafter daily, unless high levels of glycosuria are noted; blood capillary testing, by finger stab method is not required. If blood capillary levels exceed 11–13 mmol/L, the medical team must be informed and an insulin regime prescribed. These levels should subsequently be monitored 4-hourly to maintain blood glucose levels of 8–13 mmol/L.

Care must be taken to avoid the risk of hypoglycaemia in patients receiving TPN with insulin as a separate infusion. Sudden cessation of either or both infusions can create a hypoglycaemic event. The same applies if TPN is stopped and the insulin is continued. Equally, a hyperglycaemic event can occur when TPN is continued and the insulin is stopped for any reason.

Temperature, pulse and respiration

Six-hourly TPR monitoring is recommended for a patient receiving TPN. Catheter sepsis can often be detected early by nursing staff observing a sudden rise and fall in routine temperature monitoring. Central and peripheral blood cultures should be taken as soon as possible in this situation, and careful monitoring of the patient's general condition noted. Detailed recommendations for catheter sepsis management can be found in the section on complications (p. 245).

Weight

Daily weight is an important factor in patients receiving TPN. It is helpful if the gastroenterology nursing team weigh the patient at the same time each day, using the same set of scales. As discussed earlier, many malnourished patients have difficulty in excreting fluids due to reduced serum proteins and this results in an apparent weight gain. The gain is often merely excess fluid and not muscle bulk. It is only possible to rely on a patient's weight as an indicator if the fluid balance is entirely accurate on a daily basis.

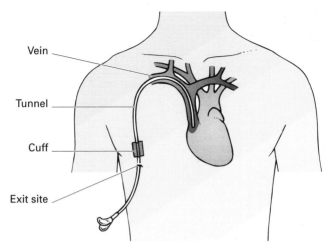

Vein

Tunnel

Cuff

Exit site

Fig 9.8 Subclavian approach to a tunnelled central line.

Dressing the line

Following the insertion of a tunnelled central line for the sole purpose of TPN, the care of the line is an important part of the gastroenterology nursing team's role. The line entry and exit sites (see Fig. 9.8) should be observed daily for any discharge, local pain or swelling. Any exudate from the line site should be assessed by the microbiology team for evidence of infection.

Care should be taken by the nursing team to support the feeding line at all times in order to reduce the risk of the line being dislodged or, in some cases, removed completely. The end of the line can be encased in sterile gauze and attached to the patient's clothing with a safety pin. Alternatively, the line can be taped to the patient's chest.

Emotional aspects

It is only to be expected that patients requiring TPN, for whatever length of time, will be anxious at the prospect of receiving nutrition in this invasive and antisocial manner. Initially, a clear and simple description of the concept of TPN may help to relieve the stress associated with this method of nutrition.

Some centres involved with TPN supply their patients with an information booklet. Diagrams illustrate the position of the feeding line and an explanation is given of the precise nursing procedures, the observations that need to be made during the period on TPN and the reasons for the detailed care regime delivered by the gastroenterology nursing team. Well-informed patients will feel more confident in the care of an experienced gastroenterology nurse who has taken time to inform them in sensitive terms of the proposed method of providing nutritional support.

Reassurance must be given to each patient commencing TPN that it is possible to reduce the period of time TPN is delivered so that administration takes place overnight.

Table 9.4 Metabolic complications

Problem	Symptoms	Possible reasons	Action
Unstable biochemistry	Consistent with abnormal serum biochemistry results (see later)	Postoperative physiological disturbances	Regular biochemical analysis
Bizarre liver function tests	Jaundice > Alkaline phosphatase > AST	Inflamed biliary tract Liver intolerant of lipid	Alteration of lipid type Consider antibiotic therapy to reduce inflammation of biliary tract
Low vitamin and trace element status	Generalised muscle weakness Dry skin and hair	Malnutrition. Disease process Disturbance of vitamin and trace element status	Prompt trace element and vitamin assessment
Sacral/ankle oedema	Swollen and painful ankles	Fluid overload Low serum albumin	Review fluid requirements Consider 20% albumin with a view to maintaining serum albumin >35 mmol/L
Negative nitrogen balance	Muscle wasting and possibly febrile following a major trauma	Hypercatabolic state induced by sepsis, trauma, inflammation	Dietitian to review patient's nutritional requirements
Dehydration	Increased urea, sodium, albumin Decreased urine output Thirst, dry skin, confusion	Pyrexia Increased fluid losses, e.g. from stoma, fistula, vomiting, diarrhoea Decreased fluid intake	Review fluid input/output Increase volume of TPN (3.0 L max.) Additional fluid (Hartman's) may be plumbed to TPN following consultation with clinical team

Table 9.4 (cont'd)

Problem	Symptoms	Possible reasons	Action
Fluid overload	Decreased urea and sodium Ankle oedema and shortness of breath	Increased fluid intake Less fluid output – lower temperature, less diarrhoea Cardiac dysfunction	Review fluid input/output Stop unnecessary fluids, Decrease volume of TPN (1.5 L min.)
Hyperglycaemia	Glycosuria Increased blood glucose , (>10 mmol/L) thirst, polyuria	Metabolic 'stress' Steroids, e.g. hydrocortisone Diabetes mellitus	Review composition, amount and rate of feed. Start sliding scale insulin
Hypolglycaemia	Low blood glucose, pallor, sweating, confusion	Hypoglycaemia Rebound hypoglycaemia Abrupt cessation of TPN	Review composition, amount and rate of feed. Check feed administrated as prescribed (no prolonged gaps). Reduce infusion rate 1–2 h prior to stopping TPN
Hypophosphataemia	Low phosphate, arrythmias, confusion, weakness, respiratory distress	Prolonged malnutrition Increased losses – renal failure, hypoparathyroidism, vitamin D deficiency	Ensure adequate phosphate repletion prior to feeding
Hyperphosphataemia	High phosphate	Excess intake. Fewer losses, e.g. renal failure, hypoparathyroidism Low vitamin D Redistribution (acidosis, tissue damage)	Review input and correct Consider amount in TPN and decrease

Table 9.4 *(cont'd)*

Problem	Symptoms	Possible reasons	Action
Hyponatraemia	Low sodium, confusion, disorientation	Reduced intake Excess water (high intake, renal failure, liver failure) Diuretic therapy	Review fluid input Review renal and hepatic function. Review diuretic therapy
Hypernatraemia	High sodium, thirst, headache	High intake Water depletion (low intake, fewer GI and renal losses, fewer insensible losses)	Review fluid balance and correct dehydration
Hypokalaemia	Low potassium Cardiac arrythmias	Reduced intake Fewer losses, e.g. renal failure, diuretics, GI secretions, liver failure, high aldosterone Redistribution, e.g. insulin, alkalosis.	Review input and correct Increase potassium in small increments
Hyperkalaemia	High potassium Cardiac arrythmias	High intake Fewer losses, e.g. renal failure, diuretics Redistribution, e.g. sepsis, tissue damage, acidosis	Review input and correct Insulin and dextrose

Many factors can cause a patient to become depressed – malnutrition, biochemical distrubance or prolonged hospital admission, perhaps due to fistulae healing. Long days, uninterrupted by meal times, will seem endless and boring. It is important that members of the nursing team recognise the signs of a depressed mood and make every effort to encourage and motivate a patient, thereby avoiding the risk of depression.

In fistula management and prolonged hospital admission, patients can be encouraged to exercise, get dressed and join their families on short outings for a change of scene away from hospital routine.

A patient who is acutely ill with gastrointestinal disease will often have no desire for food and may have difficulty in adjusting to the loss of such a basic function as eating. Anybody deprived of the comfort and pleasure of eating can develop psychological problems. As the introduction of TPN becomes established, it is often at this stage that certain patients are faced with the prospect of artificial, intravenous nutrition for the rest of their lives. This can come as a shock and present many social difficulties for both the individual and the family. With this situation to face and, in some cases, the patient's perception of a now altered body image, due to possible fistula drainage, central venous tunnelled catheter in situ, etc., one can see the advantages and support a patient would gain from an experienced and sympathetic gastroenterology nursing team.

Experience and research show that a dedicated nutritional support team including clinical nurse specialists (CNS) will enhance patient care both physically and psychologically (Hosphen 1993).

Mechanical complications associated with TPN

The mechanical complications are mainly associated with tunnelled central venous catheters.

Pneumothorax

Any patient having had a dedicated central venous feeding line inserted will require a chest X-ray to determine the position of the tip of the feeding line. An ideal position for the feeding line is at the junction of the superior vena cava and right atrium of the heart. The radiologist and medical team will determine the position of the line and should notify the gastroenterology nursing team that the line is in the correct position before TPN commences.

During radiological assessment, care should be taken by the radiologist to ensure that the patient has not suffered a pneumothorax during catheter insertion. Respiratory rate and associated pain, particularly on deep inspiration, should be carefully monitored. It is not uncommon for the initial chest X-ray to be deemed normal but for the patient to complain some hours later of shoulder tip pain and an associated cough. A further chest X-ray may reveal a pneumothorax, which, although it may be less than 20%, can potentially create problems of chest infection, pneumonia, etc. Depending on the local gastroenterological protocol, a chest drain may be necessary in cases where the pneumothorax exceeds 20%. Respiratory function should be monitored regularly and persistent chest pain reported to the medical team.

In most cases, the lung will reinflate within 2–3 days and the chest drain can then be removed. TPN can be continued throughout this period without any risk to the patient.

Catheter redirection
This event is common during insertion of a tunnelled feeding line, using a subclavian approach, when the catheter enters the jugular vein rather than the superior vena cava. The position of the line will be seen on routine chest X-ray postinsertion. Medical staff must check the position of the feeding line prior to TPN being commenced.

Uncuffed feeding lines can fall out, sometimes due to poor suturing. Experienced gastroenterology nurses will note the security of the feeding line when redressing the site and ensure the line is resutured if necessary.

Feeding line fracture or cracking
This is potentially a very serious situation which could result in air embolism or septicaemia. Whether the line is only partially cracked or entirely fractured, the proximal end of the line should be clamped immediately and the infusion of TPN stopped. The cause of damage to the catheter hub is often due to overzealous twisting of the luer locking system between the giving set and the catheter.

The repair of a catheter damaged in this way should be performed only by experienced personnel such as the CNS in TPN, or a senior member of the medical gastroenterology team. It should be remembered that, once an infusion of TPN is stopped and the patient is disconnected, the same infusion must never be reconnected for fear of contamination and possible septicaemia.

Feeding line blockage
Blockage of feeding lines can be avoided by continuous infusion of TPN. Should the infusion be interrupted for any length of time, blood will collect in the line and clot. If it is decided to deliver TPN intermittently, for instance overnight, the catheter should be 'locked' with heparinised saline 10 units/ml in order to reduce the risk of clot formation (Cottee 1995).

One reason why a feeding line may appear to be blocked is that it has become lodged against the wall of the vein. Changing the patient's position may allow it to move and become free again. If this is unsuccessful, a very gentle attempt can be made to flush sodium chloride down the line. Excessive pressure should never be used and immediate aspiration of the syringe should be implemented to ensure any small clots will be retrieved. Finally, the line should be locked with heparinised saline as above.

Very stubborn blocked lines may be treated with an antifibrinolytic agent according to local protocol, but this should only be administered by experienced medical personnel.

Any attempt to resolve a blocked line should be made by experienced staff only.

Catheter leakage
Leakage from the catheter itself can also be a serious problem with a severe risk to the patient due to sepsis and air embolism.

In this case, the infusion of TPN should be stopped and disconnected, using full aseptic technique. If the catheter is damaged, this section should be wrapped in sterile gauze and the catheter occluded above the damaged section using an atraumatic clamp, for example a Hickman crocodile non-toothed clamp. A toothed clamp will merely fracture the catheter further.

Urgent expert advice should be sought either from the CNS in TPN or an experienced member of the team. Most modern catheters can be repaired by experienced personnel.

Prevention of feeding line infections

The gastroenterology nursing team should be aware of ways in which microorganisms can enter the body via the system used for TPN. The CNS or an experienced gastroenterology nurse must demonstrate a commitment to assess and train the nursing team in the care of patients receiving nutritional support by applying specialist knowledge to the clinical setting. A protocol of care for handling the catheter and the administration equipment is essential to avoid sepsis occurring.

A simple but effective formulation of policies and guidelines must be adhered to rigidly and should incorporate the following:

- scrupulous handwashing by all disciplines involved in handling any part of the administration system
- insertion of the catheter for the administration of the nutritional support performed using a totally aseptic technique in a clean environment
- commitment from the patient's team to using the catheter solely for nutritional support
- preparation of the TPN in aseptic pharmaceutical conditions by a dedicated TPN pharmacist and team
- additions to the specially prepared bag of nutrition are not to be made at ward level
- use of a simple administration set with the minimum of additional connections
- use of three-way taps to be avoided in order to reduce risk of infection
- a new administration set to be used for each bag of TPN
- totally aseptic technique when attaching and disconnecting patients to TPN
- scrupulous and regular care and observation of the catheter site.

Catheter and site dressing

The catheter exit site may need dressing two to three times each week, making the use of an aseptic technique more significant in maintaining a low infection rate.

There has been much debate regarding dressings for the catheter used for TPN. A transparent occlusive dressing has the advantage of allowing the catheter to be clearly visible, but can cause irritation and is often difficult to remove aseptically. An adhesive gauze dressing has the disadvantage of not allowing the catheter to be visible. However, if a gauze dressing is used as well as an occlusive dressing, this ensures the security of the catheter and also allows the nurse to observe any exudate staining the gauze. Whichever dressing is chosen, an aseptic technique is very important. The cleaning solutions used most commonly for the dressing procedure contain alcohol, which is known to be effective against staphylococcus. When performing this procedure, care should be taken to clean carefully around and under the catheter at the site at which it exits from the skin.

All patients receiving TPN should have temperature, blood pressure and respiration monitored 6-hourly, particularly in the early stages of this method of nutrition. Should the patient develop a temperature, all other possible sources of infection should be considered before sepsis of the catheter is assumed. Swabs of the catheter site, wound swabs, specimens of sputum, urine and blood should all be taken, including blood cultures from the catheter plus peripheral blood cultures.

Positive blood cultures of *Staphylococcus epidermidis* or *Candida* sp. are most likely to be catheter-related, while non-catheter-related organisms are more likely to be gram-negative. In the past, there has been much controversy over whether to continue TPN after the patient has developed catheter sepsis. A popular approach suggests stopping TPN until an organism has been proven to be the cause of catheter sepsis, commencing an appropriate antibiotic therapy and instilling this in the line before flushing with sodium chloride and restarting TPN.

PERIPHERAL PARENTERAL NUTRITION

The peripheral route for the provision of nutrition to the critically ill patient offers a useful alternative in a variety of situations:

- in the event that the patient's requirement for nutritional support will not exceed 1 week and does not justify an invasive procedure
- when the hospital concerned does not have the facilities or the staff appropriately trained to prepare complex bags or to deliver the care required for central venous catheter management
- if a central venous catheter is contraindicated due to relevant veins being thrombosed
- when available sites are injured
- in the event of overwhelming sepsis
- if a patient is on renal dialysis and venous access is at a premium.

The peripheral route should not be used:

- for patients with inadequate or inaccessible peripheral veins
- for patients requiring high calcium and protein regimens that cannot be safely supplied via this route.

Due to the simplicity of peripheral nutrition, the system can be managed on a general ward, providing a more convenient method than using a short-term central venous catheter.

Practical suggestions for peripheral cannulae are as follows:

- use a long peripheral vein in the back of the hand or forearm (the larger the vein, the fewer the complications, due to larger vein size and increased blood flow)

- choose a vein that is not necessarily visible, but is palpable; these veins are secured to the surrounding tissue and not readily displaced
- avoid the large antecubital vein; this should be used only for blood sampling and should be reserved for future central catheters
- avoid veins that sit above arteries, in order to avoid formation of a fistula
- avoid veins over joints; movement will cause the cannula to bend and dislodge
- do not resort to veins in the feet for this treatment as this will immobilise the patient and give rise to an increased risk of thrombosis
- use small cannulae which do little damage to the vein but dilute vaso-irritative solution promptly.

Regimens suitable to peripheral TPN

In the past, severe restrictions were placed on peripheral TPN due to the osmolarity causing the hypertonicity of TPN solution to produce thrombotic phlebitis in small veins, whose blood flow is too low to dilute the solution rapidly. However, recently lipid has been used as the main calorie source and this lowers the osmolarity of the solution and therefore the risk of thrombotic phlebitis.

WEANING FROM TPN

The majority of patients requiring TPN will reach the point where the problem that necessitated the TPN has resolved and normal nutritional intake can be reintroduced. For many patients, this will seem a mammoth task, as they express no interest in food and thus have no appetite.

Collaboration with the dietitian will ensure that the transition from parenteral to enteral nutrition is gradual and appropriate. Large, heavy meals will be depressing and daunting for a patient who has received TPN for a long period of time. Patience and encouragement by the patient's carers are most important. Meals should be small, regular and attractively presented. Often a patient's taste will have been altered dramatically by a long period of TPN treatment. This confuses the family in their attempt to provide tasty favourites. Liquid supplement drinks provided by the dietetic department can be of help, as well as providing extra calories.

During this transition period, a food record chart is useful for the dietitian to assess the patient's calorie and protein intake. As the patient manages to tolerate increased quantities of food, so the TPN may be reduced. Patients are encouraged to tolerate 1000 kcal by mouth before TPN is reduced. This can be achieved by reducing the calorific value or by providing the normal regimen over a longer period of time – a 48-h period. The latter is probably a more structured approach.

The central venous catheter used for TPN should not be removed until the TPN team are sure that adequate nutrition will be maintained in the absence of TPN.

A final weight should be recorded on completion of TPN. At outpatient appointments, the medical team will be able to check that the patient's weight is being maintained.

SUMMARY

It is only in the last two decades that TPN has been widely accepted and the indications and disadvantages better understood. Evidence from two recent surveys into the practice of nutritional support in hospitals in the UK suggests that there is a serious lack of nutritional organisation in at least two-thirds of hospitals. Research demonstrates that poor nutritional care of patients appears to be due to the division of responsibility between departments of catering and departments of dietetics (Kings Fund 1992).

Historically, medical staff have regarded malnutrition as a nursing problem; nurses, in turn, refer nutrition problems to the dietitian. The gradual popularity and more general use of TPN, plus the known complications associated with its use, led to the formation of specialist teams in several major centres in the UK.

Following the development of specialised nutritional support teams, it was found that the adoption of strict protocols of care and the involvement of specialists with increasing experience in techniques associated with TPN considerably reduced the incidence of complications. Optimum results are more likely to be achieved when a concerted action is taken, making full use of the multidisciplinary expertise available within the NST (Payne-James 1991).

In addition to the NST meeting on a daily basis, a strong link between the departments of biochemistry, haematology and microbiology is essential to ensure accurate monitoring of patients receiving TPN.

Many patients who require HPN will find an improvement in the underlying disease that necessitated the commencement of TPN within 1 year. The longer a patient has received TPN, the more difficult the bowel finds it to adjust to enteral feeding and the transition often proves difficult. However, a patient, flexible and sensitive approach usually achieves success.

The development and advances generally seen in NSTs has meant that TPN is now an accepted and well-recognised method of providing nutrition to the malnourished patient. Experience has shown that a NST can ensure that costs are kept to a minimum and yet provide an essential, rational and comprehensive service for malnourished gastroenterological patients (Burnham 1994).

Home parenteral nutrition has been a success in the UK, with many patients being weaned from HPN in less than a year. Those remaining on HPN can enjoy a reasonable and confident quality of life with support and encouragement from the gastroenterology and nutritional support teams.

Peripheral TPN is slowly gaining in popularity in the UK, and with the wide variety of peripheral feeding lines now available, it offers the gastroenterologist the choice of a less invasive method of providing a complete nutrition regimen, without the risks involved in central venous cannulation.

The success of every patient receiving TPN depends on the attention to detail of every aspect of the process, from recognition of malnutrition to weaning from TPN back to a normal diet.

REFERENCES

Allard J P, Jeejeebhoy K N 1989 Nutritional support and therapy in the short bowel syndrome. Gastroenterology Clinics of North America 18:589–601

ASPEN Board of Directors 1993 Guidelines for the use of parenteral and enteral nutrition in adult and paediatric patients. Journal of Parenteral and Enteral Nutrition 17(4):7SA

Burnham W R 1994 The role of a nutritional support team in artificial nutritional support in clinical practice. In: Gimble G K, Payne-James J, Silk D B A (eds) Nutritional support in clinical practice. British Association of Parenteral and Enteral Nutrition. Edward Arnold, London

Buzby G P, Williford W O, Peterson O L 1988 A randomised clinical trial of total parenteral nutrition in malnourished surgical patients. Current therapy in nutrition :198–206

Cottee S 1995 Heparin lock practice in total parenteral nutrition. Professional Nurse II(1):25–26, 28–29

Dudrick S J, MacFaynen B V, Daly J M 1976 Management of inflammatory bowel disease with parenteral hyperalimentation in gastroenterological emergencies. In: Grant A, Todd E (eds) Enteral and parenteral nutrition, 2nd edn. Blackwell Scientific Publications, Oxford

Elia M 1990 Artificial nutritional support. Medicine International 82:3392–3396

Fazio V W, Coutsoftides T, Steiger E 1983 Factors influencing the outcome of treatment of small bowel cutaneous fistulae. World Journal of Surgery 7:481–488

Fleming C R 1994 Nutrition considerations in patients with Crohn's disease. Seminars in Colon and Rectal Surgery 5:167–173

Greenburgh G R, Fleming C R, Jeejeebhoy K N et al 1988 Controlled trial of bowel rest and nutritional support in the management of Crohn's disease. Gut 29:1309–1315

Griffiths A M, Ohlsson A, Sherman P M, Sutherland L R 1995 Meta-analysis of enteral nutrition as a primary treatment of active Crohn's disease. Gastroenterology 108:1056–1067

Heaton K W, Thornton J R, Emmett P M 1979 Treatment of Crohn's disease with an unrefined-carbohydrate, fibre-rich diet. British Medical Journal 2(6193):764–766

Hosphen R, Plusa S M, Kendall-Smith S et al 1993 The impact of the introduction of a clinical nutrition team in the safety and efficacy of intravenous. The pivotal role of the nutrition nurse. Procedures of the second annual meeting of the British Association of Parenteral and Enteral Nutrition

King's Fund Centre 1992 A positive approach to nutrition as treatment. Multiplex Medway, Walderslade

Larsson J, Knossan M, Er A C, Nilsson L, Thorslund S, Bjurulf P 1990 Effect of dietary supplement on nutritional status and clinical outcome in 501 geriatric patients. A randomized study. Clinical Nutrition 9(4):179–184

Lennard-Jones J E, Wood S 1991 Coping with the short bowel. Hospital Update 17(10):797–806

O'Morain C, Segal A W, Levi A J 1984 Elemental diet as primary treatment of acute Crohn's disease: a controlled trial 1984. British Medical Journal 288:1859–1862

Park L H, Duncan A, Russell R I 1990 Hypolactasia and Crohn's disease: a myth. American Journal of Gastroenterology 85(6):708–710

Payne-James J J 1991 Are nutritional teams justified? Current Medical Literature, Gastroenterology 10.2:40–43

Pirone L, Callegar C, Cornia G L, Lami F, Miglioli M, Barbara L 1988 Lactose malabsorption in adult patients with Crohn's disease. American Journal of Gastroenterology 83(11):1267–1271

Ritchie J K, Wadsworth J, Lennard-Jones J E, Rogers E 1987 Controlled multicentre therapeutic trial of an unrefined carbohydrate, fibre rice diet in Crohn's disease. British Medical Journal 295(6597):517–520

Schofield W N, Schofield C, James W P T 1985 Basal metabolic rate – review and prediction. Human Nutrition: Clinical Nutrition 39C (suppl. 1):5–96

Suarez F L, Salvaiano D A, Levitt M D 1995 A comparison of symptoms after the consumption of mild lactose-hydrolysed milk by people with self-reported severe lactose intolerance. New England Journal of Medicine 333:1–4

Thomas B (ed) 1994 Manual of diabetic practice, 2nd edn. Blackwell Scientific Publications, Oxford

FURTHER READING

Christie P M, Hill G L 1990 Effect of intravenous nutrition on nutrition and function in acute attacks of inflammatory bowel disease. Gastroenterology 99:730–736

Dalton M J, Schepers G, Gee J P et al 1984 Consultative total parenteral nutrition teams: the effect on the incidence of total parenteral nutrition related complications. Journal of Parenteral and Enteral Nutrition 8:146–152

Faubion W C, Wesley J R, Khalidi N, Silva J 1986 Total parenteral nutrition catheter sepsis: impact of the team approach. Journal of Parenteral and Enteral Nutrition 10:642–645

Grant A, Todd E 1987 Enteral and parenteral nutrition: a clinical handbook. Blackwell Scientific Publications, Oxford

Puntis J W L, Holden C E, Smallman S et al 1991 Staff training: a key factor in reducing intravascular catheter sepsis. Archives of Diseases of Childhood 66:335–337

Ryan J A, Abel R M, Abbott W M et al 1974 Catheter complication in total parenteral nutrition: a prospective study of 200 consecutive patients. New England Journal of Medicine 290:757–761

Traeger S M, Williams G B, Milliren G et al 1986 Total parenteral nutrition by a nutrition support team; improved quality of care. Journal of Parenteral and Enteral Nutrition 10:408–412

Index